SLIM FOR LIFE

SLIM FOR LIFE

MY INSIDER SECRETS TO
SIMPLE, FAST, AND LASTING
WEIGHT LOSS

Jillian Michaels

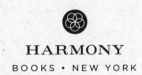

HARMONY
BOOKS · NEW YORK

Copyright © 2013 by EM Publishing, LLC

All rights reserved.
Published in the United States by Harmony Books, an imprint of the
Crown Publishing Group, a division of Random House LLC,
a Penguin Random House Company, New York.
www.crownpublishing.com

HARMONY BOOKS is a registered trademark and the circle colophon is a
trademark of Random House LLC.

Originally published in hardcover in the United States by
Harmony Books, an imprint of the Crown Publishing Group,
a division of Random House LLC, New York.

Library of Congress Cataloging-in-Publication Data
is available upon request

ISBN 978-0-385-34924-6
eBook ISBN 978-0-385-34923-9

PRINTED IN THE UNITED STATES OF AMERICA

Book design by Elizabeth Rendfleisch
Cover design by Michael Nagin
Cover photograph by Andrew MacPherson

1   3   5   7   9   10   8   6   4   2

First Paperback Edition

I'm sick of sappy book dedications. This book is not for my parents, my kids, or my "loving partner." This book is straight from me to you. It's my way for our minds to meet and have a conversation about health, hotness, and happiness. This book is dedicated to all the hot bodies out there just waiting to be transformed. Here's to you. Be awesome. Live life to the fullest. Shoot for the stars and never settle . . . an occasional compromise is okay, but *never* settle.

CONTENTS

INTRODUCTION

I have to tell you—I honestly never saw myself writing a "diet" book again. I thought I had said all there was to say about weight loss and maintenance, diet and nutrition, and even exercise. But over time I realized that maybe I and all the other "weight-loss gurus" had said too much, making things overcomplicated, confusing, even conflicting.

One expert tells you to count points, another tells you to count minute blocks, and yet another tells you to count calories. It all means the same thing on the scale, but hearing it three different ways leaves you guessing which method actually gives you better results, and which you should do. This can make a person feel overwhelmed and a little nuts. Or you have the people who *overinform* you, with information on biochemistry, kinesiology, and other science-y stuff. Once again you feel overwhelmed, and you don't understand what to do with it anyway.

The worst offenders on this shelf are out to make a quick buck with too-good-to-be-true advice. They may tell you things like "You don't really need to worry about calories to lose weight" or "You don't have to exercise to offload the fat—you can just sit still and deep breathe it away."

Bottom line, over the last several years, I've come to recognize that the more simple and straightforward I can make the information, the easier it is for you to cut through all the crap, apply the advice, and get the results you want.

So this is *Slim for Life*—a simpler, easier path.

It's a set of straightforward methods, tips, tricks, and insider secrets that pertain to diet, exercise regimen, and general lifestyle. When you follow it, it will make any weight you've been holding on to fall off quickly—and remain off!

The advice here is doable, sustainable, fast, and affordable. Life is hard enough without dreading your workout, feeling punished by your diet, or being overwhelmed by your lifestyle. Not with *Slim for Life*.

I will dispel slim myths and lay waste to dangerous weight-loss ideas that end up damaging your metabolism and setting you even farther back behind the eight ball. That's right, all that crap you've been trying, testing out, and buying into—no more. The Cookie Diet, Master Cleanse, Carb Cutting, Fat-Free, 17-Day Debacle—all over, done! This is not gimmick time. Instead, I offer you what I've found works: hundreds of straightforward ideas that are easily implemented and guaranteed to effect a dramatic body transformation.

My last promise before we get started—permanence. I've taken all I know about weight loss and distilled it into what's in this book. It offers only what works, and nothing you don't need.

The even better news is you don't have to follow all the strategies listed within these pages or follow them all the time. *Slim for Life* allows you to pick and choose what works best for you and what's manageable for your life, all while giving you better results than you imagined possible.

Slim for Life is divided into eight chapters that take into account every possible area of your life where you might hit an obstacle or have a question—Eating, Moving, At Home, On the Go—you name it, it's here. You're covered, no matter where you are or what you're doing. In any possible scenario you can imagine, I have your back and will provide you with the diet, fitness, and lifestyle advice you need to come out on top.

I've also covered every possible self-sabotaging act or slim pit-fall, from lack of support and poor self-esteem to time constraints, access issues, and financial limitations. If or when any of these issues arise, you now have a number of solutions at your fingertips with which to circumvent them all.

But it's not just about avoiding sabotage. I'll show you how to optimize your fat-burning potential and supercharge your slim with strategic advice on everything from supplementation, food combining, and meal timing to body temperature manipulation, craving crushers, slim savvy fashion tips, and much, much more.

Now that you know what you're in for, let's get down to business and deliver the changes to your body, health, and life that you've desired for so long and truly deserve.

USER'S GUIDE

As you're about to discover, there's a lot of information in this book, but none of it is meant to overwhelm you. To make sure this doesn't happen, I've created this User's Guide to illustrate how to maximize your results and personalize your plan so that you not only get the body you've always wanted, you also have no trouble keeping it.

As I mentioned, you don't have to follow *all* the recommendations in this book. Nor do you have to follow them all the time. Some are essential, and some are, well, more optional. The quantity and the quality of the tips you choose to implement will determine the quality of your results and the rate at which you achieve them.

What's the magic combination? Which tips take precedence and what percentage of them must you follow to get life-changing, body-transforming results? The simplest answer: the ones you follow regularly. I've also built in a "hierarchy of slim," which specifically tells you which pieces will give you the most bang for your weight-loss buck. It's in the form of a point system that values each piece of advice as a 3, 2, or 1: 3 is the most powerful and important, 2 is solid and useful but not utterly essential, and 1 is a helpful add-on that offers advice on how to implement your slim lifestyle. All will help you get your slim on—so if you like one more than the other, have at it. That's the whole point of this book: structuring what works for you and your life.

At the end of each chapter is a checklist where you'll check off the ideas you can realistically see yourself incorporating into your life—permanently. Then in Chapter 8, our final chapter and wrap-up, I will assess your total slim score aggregate from all the preceding chapters and tell you exactly what it means to you and for your results. Once you've totaled up your points, I'll make recommendations for you based on the category range you fall in. If necessary, we'll up the ante by fine-tuning your tip selection (both quality and quantity) to make sure you succeed.

Choose the strategies you like most, while utilizing your knowledge of which tips take weight-loss precedence, and you'll have all you need to help you select, organize, optimize, and implement a personalized action plan that will deliver fast results and last forever.

Be aware, while there are universal laws of slim that apply to us all equally (they tend to be biochemically focused information about food and fitness), many strategies in *Slim for Life* will affect some of us more powerfully than others. (These are often more behaviorally focused suggestions on topics like building support and gearing your environment for success.)

Here's my suggestion: as you read through each chapter, note the number next to each tip. The tips that I've given a 3 rating (the power tips) are all top priority. Do anything and everything you can to follow them and check them off in the checklist at the end of each chapter. For the tips that I've given a 1 or 2 rating to, picture yourself implementing them as you read the chapter. Ask yourself, "Are they realistic to my lifestyle? Do they seem doable to me?" Obviously the ones that do, you should check off as well. The ideas you aren't sure about, I want you to put to the test. Try a couple each week. See how they work for you. Were they difficult to implement? Were they effective? This is literally how you determine what works and what doesn't for *you*, so you can permanently change your behaviors for the better.

Put the tips to which you have an immediate "no way in hell" reaction out of your mind for now. Chances are, if your aversion to them is that strong, and they feel impossible or ridiculous to you, it doesn't matter how effective they might be—you won't employ them. Guess what? There's a good chance you won't have to. It's likely you'll rack up enough slim changes that the tips you can't manage will be irrelevant. When we get to Chapter 8 and you add up your slim score and are looking for more radical results, then we'll revisit your rejected tips with a more open mind. Worry about that when we get there.

Now, fair warning, there's some information here that you won't be rewarded points for. Here's why: even though they're great tips and I want you to employ them, they don't *directly impact* your actual weight loss. Instead they facilitate it. So, for example, tips for saving money on healthy eating and exercising and dressing in slimming ways will not be awarded a point rating as they're optional and have no direct impact on the scale. They will, however, smooth the way to slim and make your life better overall, so I highly recommend you implement them. Getting and living slim is really about the whole picture after all, right?

By the way, there will be a few tips in here that don't reinvent the wheel—you've likely heard them before. I debated whether to include the ones that are more commonly known, as I always strive to give you the most current and cutting-edge information, but I ended up arriving at the conclusion that I must. Here's why: first, all of you have varying levels of knowledge on the subject matter of slim. On the off chance that you're new to the topics of diet and fitness entirely, I didn't want to rob you of Slim 101. Second, I worried that if you didn't see the basic or old-hat information listed in these chapters, you might think It wasn't important—but it is. In addition to teaching you new state-of-the-art slim strategies, I'm also going to improve upon any existing knowledge you may have of the more common weight-loss methods by explaining to you *why* the advice is important and *how* to better implement it into your life.

Now, let's roll.

CHAPTER 1

EATING

The purpose of this chapter is to lay your *foundation* for lifelong control over your weight, and that starts with what you eat. You'll see that this and the exercise chapter are some of the longest ones in the book—that's on purpose. These two subject matters are the cornerstones of successful weight loss. And it's my goal to teach you how to master and implement them in the easiest and most effective ways possible.

I've always hated the word *easy*, because I truly believe that nothing in life worth having is easy, *but* my goal here is to make your relationship with food and eating healthy easier—as easy as *possible*. In other words, there might be some sacrifice, but I've done my best to make it as effortless and painless as can be.

Slim for Life's effectiveness relies on applying the proven science behind fast and lasting weight loss to your daily life. It's all digested throughout these pages into strategies, tips, tricks, and "secrets" that allow you to lose weight without needing a mind-numbing education in biochemistry, tediously counting calories, or wasting hours in the gym. The lifestyle changes I'm suggesting ultimately will help you burn the most calories as quickly as possible without making you miserable and bored.

....

Cracking the Diet Code

SLIM CALORIE HABITS

LIVE IN THE RED • • • 3 POINTS

The term *red* has a negative connotation when it comes to finances, but when it comes to calories and weight loss, it's key. You simply must burn more calories in a day than you consume. This book is designed to help you do this without hours of calorie counting and calculating.

Fat is nothing more than stored energy; a calorie is a unit of energy. The energy you don't use gets stored in your body as fat. The obvious way to lose weight, despite whatever load of crap the diet charlatans tell you, is to eat less and move more. But that's not always as simple as it sounds, is it?

We used to believe, until very recently, that we could calculate weight loss based on a simple equation: a pound equals 3,500 calories, so we need to create a 3,500-calorie deficit to lose a pound. For example, if you have 25 pounds to lose, then based on the 3,500-calorie theory, if you exercise and reduce your diet for a combined deficit of 1,000 calories a day, you should lose 25 pounds in about 12 weeks (2 pounds per week). The most current research, however, published in 2011 in *The Lancet*, suggests that this rule of thumb is both a misnomer and misleading. Not only do some people lose weight faster than others, but the amount that people lose is not equal within the same time frame.

The researchers in this study suggest that there are other factors at play that we hadn't previously thought were relevant—age, height, weight, gender, body fat percentage, and resting metabolic rate. These count when it comes to estimating a truer calculation of calories used versus those taken in each day.

To see what it will take you to lose weight calorie-wise in conjunction with the amount of activity you're willing to put in, the researchers have created a mathematical tool, available to the public online: http://bwsimulator.niddk.nih.gov/. You simply go to this page and enter your personal info and the amount and intensity of training you're willing to do, and the simulator will ballpark for you how much you should be eating in a day. Try it—it's supercool. I used it during Season 14 with our *Biggest Loser* contestants, and it worked like a charm.

In the event you want to go a little more old school, we can get in the ballpark of what you're burning in a day right now with a pen and paper and a calculator. The first thing we'll do is calculate your basal metabolic rate (BMR), the amount of calories your body uses for involuntary bodily functions—basically when you're asleep or at rest. Your BMR doesn't take into account the number of calories you burn from your daily activity, though. That's your AMR, or active metabolic rate. I'll get to that in a minute.

The **BMR formula** uses the variables of height, weight, age, and gender to calculate the body's energy expenditure. The only factors it omits are lean body mass (the ratio of muscle to fat that a body has) and biochemistry. If you have hypothyroid, polycystic ovary

SLIM MYTH:
Genetics make you fat.
FAST FACT: Although it may be harder for you to maintain slim than it is for that friend who eats whatever he or she wants and never gains an ounce, you're not relegated to obesity because of your genetics. I've never met a person I couldn't help take the weight off. People nevertheless embrace this theory for weight-loss failure. Genetics are dynamic, not static. This means that we affect the expression of our genes through our lifestyle choices. Stop comparing yourself to others. I guarantee that if you eat well, move more, and take care of yourself, you'll be slim and healthy.

syndrome (PCOS), insulin resistance, or estrogen dominance, there's no way for the BMR formula to read that—you need blood work and an endocrinologist to deal with these issues. Barring a hormonal disorder, however, this formula will be fairly accurate overall. One additional caveat: for very muscular people, it will slightly underestimate the calorie burn, and for those with a higher percentage of body fat, it will slightly overestimate it.

Use the following BMR formula for your gender to calculate your BMR:

Women: BMR = 655 + (4.35 x weight in pounds) + (4.7 x height in inches) - (4.7 x age in years)

Men: BMR = 66 + (6.23 x weight in pounds) + (12.7 x height in inches) - (6.8 x age in years)

After you've run through these simple calculations and come up with your BMR, we need to then calculate your AMR. This next exercise is going to tell us how many calories you're burning in a day *without* adding in your exercise burn—simply the amount you burn in an average day of your life (sans exercise).

Identify which category you fall into:

1. If you're chained to your desk and sedentary most of your day, you're a 1.1. People who fall into this category would be receptionists, telemarketers, and customer service reps.

2. If you're mildly active over the course of your day, you're a 1.2. People who fall into this category are housewives and retail salespeople—basically folks who are on their feet throughout the day but not exerting themselves as a part of their job (though the moms among you might argue with me on this one).

3. If you're active and on your feet moving at a fast pace, you're a 1.3. I fall into this category, as most trainers will. So will a plumber or an electrician. This applies to those who are up, moving, and exerting energy but not working on a chain gang.

4. If you're extremely physically active, you're a 1.4. Construction workers, professional athletes, essentially anyone who is constantly exerting themselves throughout the course of their day fits into this group.

Once you've identified which category fits you best, take that number and multiply it by your BMR. So if my BMR is 1,300, I would multiply it by 1.3 and arrive at 1,690. Now I know that if I eat around 1,700 calories a day on the days I don't work out, I won't gain weight. Additionally, on the days I do work out, I'll be able to factor in that additional burn and ramp up my AMR. Let's say I add an hour of training and I burn 500 calories during that hour, then my total AMR will be 2,300.

With all the info I've just given you here, there's absolutely no way you won't be able to figure out your personal magic number. Use the URL from earlier in this section to calculate your weight-loss goals (the amount of weight you want to lose and the time frame you want to lose it in), and it will tell you how many calories you should be taking in daily. Or use the AMR equation I've provided here. As long as you don't eat over your AMR on a daily basis, you won't gain weight.

GET THE LOWDOWN • • • 3 POINTS

If you don't want to do any math and just want a bottom-line number for accelerated weight loss, here it is: 1,200 calories a day if you're a woman and 1,600 if you're a man. Don't go any lower than that. Anything less will leave you miserable, hungry, and weak and possibly cause your body to cannibalize its own muscle tissue. Ultimately you won't have to count your calories at all after you get used to following *Slim for Life,* as the tips in this book, when applied, will healthfully regulate your food intake without you even realizing it. *It's important to know the basics, though, as these principles are going to be the foundation of your new slimming lifestyle.*

CLEAR OUT THE KITCHEN CABINETS • • • 3 POINTS

This is always my first step when I help people get slim. I go through their cabinets, fridge, and pantry and dump out the fattening junk foods. You can't eat what's not there.

DOWNSIZE: SWITCH TO "SLIM-SIZE" PORTIONS • • • 3 POINTS

Ever heard the maxim *less is more*? This should be a no-brainer when it comes to food—it's an easy way to seriously cut calories *without* cutting out the foods you love, without feeling deprived. If there's a smaller version of the food you're purchasing and consuming, buy it. Just in case you're clueless as to what I mean, here are some examples. When ordering out, always ask for the smallest size, or baby portion, available. Get the small order of fries, the child-size ice cream cup, the Tall-size mocha at Starbucks. Choose the cheeseburger instead of the triple-patty bacon extravaganza. Get it? The same is true when you're grocery shopping: buy the mini-bagels, the baby muffins, and the 4-ounce yogurt container, not the 6-ounce. Even choosing a smaller piece of fruit will reduce the sugar content you consume, as well as the calories. This simple portion-control tactic will reduce your calorie intake with minimal effort and thought.

WRITE IT DOWN, ADD IT UP • • 2 POINTS

This one can be so tedious, especially when you're on the go. But the reason we health folks say it all the time is that tracking your intake helps you eat less. It forces you to stop and figure out how much you're actually eating, it helps you realize when you're graz-ing too much, and it allows you to tally up your calories at the end of the day. As time consuming as it is to do, study after study on successful long-term weight loss pinpoints the fact that daily, accurate journaling (leaving nothing out, even binge days) is *the* key ingredient to keeping the pounds off. According to a six-month study of 1,685 dieting individuals, published in the *American Jour-nal of Preventive Medicine,* those who tracked their food daily kept off as much as twice the weight as those who tracked it one day a week or less.

Here's the secret part that no one tells you: you don't have to do it forever. I don't even remember the last time I actually wrote my food down. Now, if you like to keep an ongoing log, then God bless, but there are only three situations when I really need you to buckle down and track in this way: (1) right now, for the first two weeks, as you begin to get your slim on, so you can get a sense of what you're eating each day; (2) when you're successfully losing or maintaining and you add a new food to your usual repertoire; and (3) if your weight plateaus.

We really are creatures of habit, and our food choices show it. Did you know that most people eat only twenty foods consistently, out of the thousands of foods available? By tracking your food at the beginning, you'll learn how to account for the number of calo-ries in the foods you're regularly eating, as well as create awareness of your eating habits and grazing patterns.

Think about it. I bet you have the same three or four things for breakfast every day, eat the same three or four things for lunch, and hit the same three to five restaurants for dinner. I know I do. I'm pretty sure you also purchase the same brand of bread, turkey, cheese, yogurt, and oatmeal—just as I do. Because I eat so many of the same things, I know there are 80 calories in an egg, 100 calories in my Oikos low-fat vanilla Greek yogurt, and 80 calories in my Horizon organic low-fat cheese stick. I also know that my two-eggs-over-easy breakfast with two slices of dry Ezekiel toast equals roughly 360 calories.

I don't need to food-journal anymore, because I know exactly how much I'm eating. I've previously added it up.

Now, addressing point number two: if a new restaurant opens up in town and you add its pasta Florentine to your regular dinner lineup, I don't need you to start writing all your food down again, but I do need you to take a stab at figuring out roughly how many calories are in this new addition to see if it makes a significant difference in your calorie intake. If the calorie count is not listed on the menu, ask the waitress what's in it and how it's prepared, which should point you in the right direction. Once you know, you can reconfigure what you're eating overall if necessary to make sure you don't overeat. Again, you'll need to do it only once. I'm sure you'll remember for the next time.

Last, if you've plateaued, the very first thing you should do is start logging your daily food intake again—for three days, to be exact. Often people come to me, tearing their hair out, protesting "I've plateaued—the scale has completely screeched to a halt." In a few rare occasions this is possible, and I'll tell you how to manage it later on in the book, but weight loss stalls usually because people have been eating too much (or even too little) and just don't realize it. By examining exactly *how much* food you've been eating for three days, you'll be able to quickly get to the bottom of things.

If you're wondering how to figure out the calories in a certain food or meal when it doesn't have a label, there are plenty of apps, pocket calorie-counting books, and websites that will allow you to do it easily. I know because I created one of each. If you aren't a fan of JillianMichaels.com, my Slim-down Solution app, or my pocket calorie-counting book (hard to imagine, I know, but on the extreme off chance), there are plenty of others out there that will help you get the job done.

BAG IT • • 2 POINTS

Never eat out of a big, *bottomless* bag—it can lead to unadulterated, mindless eating and sometimes may add up to your entire daily calorie requirement. (Check out the calories in a bag of tortilla chips. A 7.5-ounce bag equals about 1,039 calories—without adding in the guacamole calories.) This said, bagging it *can* be a good thing when it comes to snacking and portion control. Simply dole out your allotted portion from a big bag into smaller snack-size Baggies so they're calorie controlled, then grab and go. Plus, many companies now make snacking bags just the right size to hold 100–150 calorie snacks. There are a lot of prepackaged items that measure 100 calories.

BABY-STEP YOUR WAY TO FEWER CALORIES • • 2 POINTS

Consistent, daily calorie cutbacks are a positive and effective way to baby-step yourself into even bigger calorie savings over the long term. Try this: save 100 calories per day for a year. It's easier than you might imagine.

What is 100 calories equal to?

14 potato or corn chips
1 (8.2-ounce) can of soda
4.3 ounces white wine
8 ounces beer
1½ tablespoons ranch salad dressing
2½ Oreo sandwich cookies
3 tablespoons of Ben & Jerry's Chocolate Chip Cookie Dough
    Ice Cream
1.1 ounces McDonald's french fries (kid's portion)

These easy eliminations can remove 10 to 12 unwanted pounds in a year. Not bad, huh? For more ideas on how to do this when you're eating out, see the quick and easy calorie cuts that I've sprinkled throughout this book.

EAT REAL

DISCRIMINATE—DON'T ELIMINATE • • • 3 POINTS

Don't cut out major food groups or macronutrients like carbs, fats, meat, or grains. Every time someone wants to write a new diet book, they try to reinvent the wheel, and one of the key ways they do that is by playing with the macronutrient ratio of meals or cutting out a particular type of food. I know you know what I'm talking about, and I'm willing to bet you've experimented with at least one of these diet fads, like low-carb, fat-free, or paleo, to name just a few. Here's the deal. Fats, carbs, and protein all play necessary roles in the way our bodies function. We need them—yes, fat too. And a fat-free diet can increase your cravings. Fat is an essential element and should make up 20 to 30 percent of your daily food intake. You can choose fats that support your health and immune system, like salmon, coconut oil, avocados, and nuts.

The key is to eat quality, more nutritious versions of the macronutrients and food groups. That will serve another purpose, too—to keep you full longer. Try *substituting* a high-protein, high-fiber grain like quinoa (pronounced KEEN-wah) for white rice, which is nutrient empty; grab olive oil, which is a healthy fat, rather than hydrogenated trans fats. Reach for grass-fed, natural beef, not corn-fed meat laden with hormones and antibiotics.

SLIM MYTH:
High-protein/low-carbohydrate diets are a healthy way to lose weight.
FAST FACT: Complex carbs are a necessary source of essential vitamins and minerals that the body needs for normal hormonal balance, a healthy reproductive system, and good skin, nails, hair growth, and eyesight. In addition, eating fewer than 130 grams of carbohydrates a day can lead to something called ketosis, which is a buildup of ketones (partially broken-down fats) in your blood. Ketosis can cause your body to produce high levels of uric acid, which is a risk factor for gout (a painful swelling of the joints) and kidney stones. Remember, fat comes from too many calories, not from too many carbs.

I'll get into this more later, but the point is to eat with common sense and balance. And you don't need to make yourself miserable because a diet says you can never have a sandwich again. As long as you eat quality food and make sure to get a good balance of healthy proteins, fats, and carbs every day, you'll be fine. Here are some examples of what meals or snacks might look like:

BREAKFAST

Oatmeal with crushed walnuts; or

Tomato, spinach, and mushroom omelet with whole-grain
toast; or

Low-fat Greek yogurt with fresh fruit

LUNCH

Grilled fish tacos with a corn tortilla and side of brown rice; or

BBQ chicken breast with a side of quinoa; or

Grass-fed burger on
a whole-grain bun
with a mixed green
salad

> **EZ CALORIE CUT**
> Order a naked salad without croutons.
> **CUT: 120 CALORIES** (1 ounce = 20 croutons)

SNACK

Celery sticks with almond butter; or

Hummus with veggie sticks; or

Organic low-fat cheese stick and apple slices

DINNER

Chicken fajitas made with olive oil and a side of black beans; or

Pork chop with baked brussels sprouts and beet salad; or

Grilled skirt steak with tomato and mozzarella salad

DON'T EAT CHEMICAL CRAP • • • 3 POINTS

As I briefly mentioned in my "Don't discriminate" tip, you should aim to eat quality, nutritionally dense food, which will nourish your body, boost your immunity, fight the aging process, and burn fat. Don't be surprised—it can taste great, too. I don't expect you to lead a life of treat abstinence, though. I get it if you have some sugar or, God forbid, some white flour from time to time. I just don't want these foods to comprise the majority of your calorie intake. When you consume them occasionally as a smaller part of a healthy diet and lifestyle, they won't do much harm.

Where I want you to be diligent is with fake food—frankenfood. Do your best to never, *ever* consume food with chemical additives— the unpronounceable crap that goes into heavily processed foods for a variety of reasons, most of which are related to cost.

Now, if you're wondering what this has to do with being skinny, the answer is simple—many chemicals added to food can make you fat. In my line of work, we refer to these ingredients as obe-sogens. They can make you sick, too, but for the specific purposes of this book, the metabolic damage is our primary concern. Your metabolism is essentially your personal biochemistry that, among many other things, regulates your hormone balance *and* your body weight. Chemicals in our food disrupt the body's biochemistry and throw off metabolic function. They literally incite a war in the body, activating it to make more fat cells, store more fat, and create cancer, heart disease, autoimmune problems, and a host of other issues of which we are just starting to become aware.

HERE IS MY TOP-TEN MUST-AVOID-WHENEVER-POSSIBLE LIST:

1. Trans fat, aka hydrogenated oils. Trans fats, used to enhance and extend the shelf life of food products, are among the most dangerous substances you can consume. They're often found in deep-fried fast foods and certain processed foods made with margarine or partially hydrogenated vegetable oils. Numerous studies show that trans fats increase LDL ("bad") cholesterol levels while decreasing HDL ("good") cholesterol; they increase the risk of heart attacks, heart disease, and strokes; and they contribute to increased inflammation, diabetes, and other health problems.

Found in: any vegetable oil that has been hydrogenated (hydrogenated soybean oil, hydrogenated safflower oil, etc.), margarine, chips and crackers, baked goods, and most fast foods.

2. High-fructose corn syrup (HFCS), or corn sugar. High-fructose corn syrup is a highly refined sweetener that many believe has become the number-one source of calories in America. It's found in almost all processed foods. Based on current research, it's a safe bet that HFCS packs on the pounds faster than any other ingredient, while it also increases LDL ("bad") cholesterol levels, and contributes to the development of obesity, diabetes, and tissue damage, among other harmful effects.

Found in: soft drinks, most processed foods, breads, candy, flavored yogurts, salad dressings, canned vegetables, and cereals.

3. Artificial sweeteners (sucralose, aspartame, and saccharin). Pretty much any sweetener you find in a small blue, yellow, or pink packet should be avoided. These chemicals are known to be neurotoxins and carcinogens. They're believed to account for more adverse reactions than all other foods and food additives combined. Studies have shown that these chemicals cause sugar cravings and can train your body to be unable to recognize true sugar calories, which can cause obesity. The two main ingredients of aspartame, phenylalanine and aspartic acid, stimulate the release of insulin, a hormone that instructs your body to store fat. A large dose of phenylalanine can decrease serotonin levels. Serotonin is the neurotransmitter that tells you when you're full. Low levels of serotonin can increase cravings, which can lead to weight gain.

Also known to erode intelligence and affect short-term memory, these artificial sweeteners may lead to a wide variety of ailments including brain tumors; diseases like lymphoma, diabetes, multiple sclerosis, Parkinson's, Alzheimer's, fibromyalgia, and chronic fatigue; emotional disorders like depression and anxiety attacks; dizziness, headaches, nausea, mental confusion, migraines, and seizures.

Found in: most diet or sugar-free foods, including soda, desserts, sugar-free gum, beverage mixes, baking goods, sweeteners, cereals, breath mints, even chewable vitamins and toothpaste.

4. Artificial colors (Red no. 40, Yellow no. 6, Blue nos. 1 and 2). Food coloring has been linked to everything from ADHD to chromosomal damage to thyroid cancer. Your thyroid is critical to your metabolic function, and anything that attacks the thyroid is extremely bad for your waistline and, obviously, your overall health. There are many natural ways to color foods: beets have been used for red, turmeric has been used for yellow, carrots have been used for orange, spinach for green, and purple cabbage for blue and purple to name a few.

Found in: candy, beverages, cereal, cheese, bakery products, and ice cream.

5. Sodium nitrites and nitrates. Both these food additives (which are fairly close cousins; the only difference is that nitrates have one more oxygen atom than nitrites) are used as preservatives and flavoring in bacon, ham, hot dogs, luncheon meats, corned beef, smoked fish, and other processed meats. Nitrites are also used to color food. Both ingredients are highly carcinogenic once they enter the human digestive system. There they form nitrosamine compounds that enter the bloodstream and wreak havoc on the internal organs, the liver and pancreas in particular. Why should you care

about the pancreas? Because it's directly responsible for insulin production, a key hormone in successful weight management. (Right
when you think I'm worried only about your health, I prove I can
multitask and simultaneously worry about your waistline.) Sodium
nitrite is widely regarded as a toxic ingredient, and the USDA actually tried to ban it in the 1970s, but food manufacturers vetoed it,
complaining they had no alternative for preserving packaged meat
products. Why does the industry still use this chemical? Simple:
it turns meats bright red. It's a color fixer, and it makes old, dead
meats appear fresh and vibrant.

Found in: hot dogs, bacon, ham, luncheon meat, cured meats,
corned beef, smoked fish, and any other type of processed meat.

6. Growth hormones (rBST, rBGH). Artificial hormones are given to
conventionally raised dairy cows and cattle and put in their feed.
This is done either to boost their milk production or to fatten them
up for slaughter at an extremely accelerated pace. Studies have
linked the human consumption of these hormones to both obesity
and early puberty.

Found in: nonorganic dairy products and meats.

7. Monosodium glutamate (MSG). MSG is an amino acid used as a
flavor enhancer in soups, salad dressings, chips, frozen entrees, and
many restaurant foods. It's a known excitotoxin, a substance that
overexcites brain cells in the hypothalamus to the point of damage
or death. The hypothalamus, located just above the brain stem, is
responsible for certain metabolic processes as well as activities of
the autonomic nervous system.

Why is this important? One of the most important functions of
the hypothalamus is to connect the nervous system to the endocrine system via the pituitary gland. The hypothalamus controls,
among many other things, hunger. Ever wonder why, when you

eat food that contains MSG, it's hard to stop eating? This might be the answer. Studies have shown that MSG affects the neurological pathways of the brain, disengaging the "I'm full" function and causing increased hunger and strong food cravings. In addition, regular consumption of MSG may result in myriad adverse side effects, including depression, disorientation, eye damage, fatigue, headaches, and obesity. Don't be fooled if you don't see it as a listed ingredient—MSG is very often camouflaged under the guise of sodium caseinate, hydrolyzed yeast, hydrolyzed vegetable protein, or autolyzed yeast.

Found in: Chinese takeout and restaurant foods (ask to hold the MSG), many snacks, chips, cookies, seasonings, soup products, canned foods, frozen dinners, and lunch meats.

8. Butylated hydroxyanisole (BHA) and butylated hydroxytoluene (BHT). BHA and BHT are preservatives commonly found in most nonorganic cereals, chewing gum, potato chips, and vegetable oils. They are oxidants that keep foods from changing color, changing flavor, or becoming rancid. They primarily affect the neurological system of the brain, which can alter behavior, disrupt your endocrine system (hormones), and form cancer-causing reactive compounds in your body, potentially leading to cancer. It may be hard to find packaged products without BHA or BHT, but you can find them—make sure you read the labels carefully. It's definitely worth it to try.

Found in: potato chips, gum, cereal, frozen sausages, enriched rice, lard, shortening, candy, and Jell-O.

9. Antibiotics. Antibiotics are routinely given to farm animals to fight infections from inhumane feedlot conditions and to cause the animals to grow larger and faster than normal. For all you pescatarians out there who think you're safe, antibiotics (along with pesticides for sea lice—yuk!) are also given to farm-raised fish for the same reasons.

In case you haven't figured out where I'm going with this, antibiotics don't just affect the animals that ingest the drugs; they also affect the humans who eat the animals. A number of studies suggest that the overuse of antibiotics may be greatly contributing to our expanding waistlines, causing people to pack on fat like farm animals. There are many suspected reasons for why this is happening. Low and steady doses of antibiotics can cause "unusual" activity in genes that are linked to breaking down carbohydrates and regulating cholesterol (blood fat) levels. Antibiotics also kill the "good bacteria" in our gut, which help us to absorb vitamins and minerals. If we can't absorb these micronutrients, then we can't effectively synthesize hormones.

The list of possible concerns is endless. For more in-depth details on antibiotics and how they wreak havoc with weight, read the "Drugs That Sabotage Your Slim" section of Chapter 3. Beyond contributing to obesity, the overuse and ingestion of antibiotics is causing a massive threat to humanity by creating "superbugs," or bugs that are resistant to antibiotics, like MRSA. Their overuse is also linked to yeast infections, leaky gut syndrome, candida, and more. You can avoid unintentionally taking them by going organic with your meat and eating wild-caught fish as often as possible.

Found in: conventionally raised livestock (including poultry) and farm-raised fish.

10. Pesticides. A study conducted by the Mercer University School of Medicine examined whether pesticide exposure plays a role in worldwide childhood obesity. The researchers observed nearly 6,800 subjects aged six to nineteen. They determined individuals' exposure to environmental pesticides through the use of urine tests, so they could identify the concentrations of pesticide residues. They found a higher prevalence of obesity in the participants with high urinary concentrations of a pesticide known as 2.5-dichlorophenol (2.5-DCP). Why should you care about this hard-to-pronounce stuff? It's simple: *2.5-DCP is one of the most widely used pesticides on the planet.* Now, this particular study focused on kids, but many other studies have found similar effects with adults. Pesticides disrupt the endocrine system, which in turn causes the metabolism to "malfunction." And you know where that leads—right to your bottom (or your belly).

Found in: the majority of nonorganic fruits and vegetables.

LAND, SEA, OR TREE •• 2 POINTS

If it didn't come from the ground or the ocean or have a mother—don't eat it. Think about it. Twinkies and Cheetos—what the hell are these? There's no Twinkie tree, and I'm pretty positive that nothing ever gave birth to a Cheeto. This goes back to what I was saying earlier about chemicals in food. Foods that don't have an obvious organic origin are pure chemicals, and as we've established, chemicals make us fat. Following this tip is an easy way to identify obesogens without doing a ton of label reading and ingredient Googling. If it doesn't come from nature, don't eat it.

GO BACK TO NATURE •• 2 POINTS

Don't be derivative. Eat real versions of the food you're choosing to consume. Have a baked sweet potato, not a frozen bag of sweet potato fries. Have a bowl of berries or mash them into a fruit spread, not Smucker's jam, which also contains high-fructose corn syrup, a big NO here! Air-pop popcorn kernels instead of eating bagged popcorn (with butter). Have an actual piece of cheese, not Cheese

---

EZ CALORIE CUT

Instead of drinking an 8-ounce chocolate milk shake, drink a fruit-only smoothie.

CUT: 280 CALORIES

Whiz from a can filled with preservatives. Get the idea? Basically, when you go to eat something, first ask yourself whether the food is in its most natural, unprocessed form. If it isn't, swap it out for "whole" food. Why am I being so adamant here? Because these derivatives of the real deal are overly processed and usually contain tons of extra calories and chemicals that are making us fat. It's pretty simple to say no to the fake stuff when you know what's in it.

KEEP IT CLEAN • • 2 POINTS

I think you may have gleaned this already, but on the extremely off chance that you didn't: go organic whenever possible. As I've said, the pesticides, hormones, and antibiotics in our foods are making us sick *and fat*. I realize that times are tough, but the good news is that not everything has to be organic.

Here's where you should prioritize your organic dollars: beef, dairy, ocean-caught seafood, and thin-skinned fruits and vegetables. If you can find a way to come up with an extra twenty bucks a week for groceries (and use the tips in Chapter 6 to save money on food), I promise, you can make a huge impact on your health, your weight, and ultimately your pocketbook. That's right—spending a bit more now will save you a fortune later. Sickness is expensive. In fact, it's the number-one cause of bankruptcy in America today.

HERE ARE THE TWELVE "DIRTIEST" FRUITS AND VEGGIES.
YOU SHOULD CONSUME THESE "DIRTY DOZEN" ONLY IF
THEY'RE ORGANIC:

Apples	Nectarines
Bell peppers	Peaches
Celery	Pears
Cherries	Potatoes
Grapes (imported)	Spinach
Lettuce	Strawberries

Conversely, other fruits and veggies have less pesticide residue, so you don't need to spend your hard-earned dollars on organic. They have either a thick skin or natural insecticides that protect them from pests without chemicals.

HERE IS A LIST OF FRUITS AND VEGGIES YOU MAY HAVE HEARD REFERRED TO AS THE "CLEAN FIFTEEN":

Asparagus	Mango
Avocado	Onions
Cabbage	Pineapple
Cantaloupe	Sweet onions
Corn	Sweet peas
Eggplant	Sweet potatoes/yams
Grapefruit	Watermelon
Kiwi fruit	

If you can't afford or don't have access to an organic version of any of the Dirty Dozen, swap that choice out with an option from the Clean Fifteen. For example: have a mango instead of an apple. Have a grapefruit instead of berries. And though it's not on this list, if you can't afford organic milk, try coconut milk or almond milk instead. They don't have added hormones or antibiotics in them.

FORGET ABOUT FAT-FREE •• 2 POINTS

I'm sure that at some point in your life, even if not right now, you've fallen for the fat-free-food phenomenon. Beware—just because the label says it's fat-free doesn't mean it's free of calories or good for you. Fat-free foods often add in fillers and chemical crap to make up for the lack of taste, nutrients, texture, and palatability. Make sure you do more than glance at the label. You'll likely find that it lists HFCS, modified food starch, sugar, salt, and a host of chemicals, food colorings, and preservative agents. That doesn't sound free to me. The costs will be plenty to your health and waistline. Ideally, you'll choose the low-fat version. I'd even prefer you choose a full-fat version over heavily processed nonfat options.

MAXIMIZE YOUR NUTRIENTS

EAT IN TECHNICOLOR •• 2 POINTS

Following this simple guideline will yield great results: *White food = bad. Colorful food = good.* To clarify, processed, white food is bad (white pasta, white bread, non-whole-grain cereals, white rice, and the like)—basically, anything that comes from white, bleached flour that's been stripped of fiber and nutrients. These foods are nutritional wastelands. They can be high in calories, and they send your blood sugar skyrocketing, which is bad, bad, bad for weight loss. White fish, egg whites, chicken breasts are all fine; these are "healthy whites." And conversely, food that's colored *naturally* is great for you. Deeply colorful berries, apples, citrus, and dark greens are loaded with powerful phytonutrients and fiber that help to boost fat metabolism, fight aging, improve immunity, spur energy, and control hunger. The more color on your plate, the better!

GO LOCAL • 1 POINT

Follow the hundred-mile rule. Whenever possible, eat food that's been grown within one hundred miles of where you live. First, it supports the local economy and helps to decentralize the food system, which is really important as big food companies are infiltrating every aspect of our lives and making us fat with processed junk. Second, eating locally saves you money on groceries, because the local farmers in your area don't have the overhead that supermarket

SLIM MYTH:

Vegetarian diets are healthier than meat-eating ones.

FAST FACT: Sure, eating lots of veggies is healthy. But as I've said before, cutting out an entire "real" food group is a bad idea. We're omnivores; we've evolved to eat both animal proteins and plants. Animal products contain key nutrients like iron, B vitamins, omega-3s, and calcium, which are critical for your health. While you can find plant-based foods with *some* of these nutrients, the amounts are often significantly smaller.

Just because you're vegan doesn't mean you're healthy. You could still be eating tons of processed grains, soy, sugar, and chemicals—which are not good food choices. The key is to eat lots of healthy, organic veggies, 100 percent whole grains, wild-caught fish, and grass-fed, unprocessed meat in moderation.

chains do for marketing, transport, and employees, as well as the real estate costs of a storefront.

Third—and most important where this book is concerned—local food is fresher. Locally grown fruits and veggies are better for you because they've been given time to ripen naturally (conventional produce is often picked before it's ripe, then is sprayed to look pretty), allowing the nutrients that occur in the plant to mature. Also, when fruits and vegetables travel long distances, they oxidize, which means they age en route and lose powerful nutrients and antioxidants. Remember, good nutrition is a critical component of your overall health and immunity as well as your weight management, as it helps to optimize hormone balance and metabolic function.

You can get meat, cheese, and eggs from local farmers as well. It's better for the environment and local economy, and to find out if it's better for your waistline, too, make sure to ask them if they use hormones or antibiotics on any of their animals. If they do, this purchase is no better for your *weight* than store-bought versions of the same items. Almost always, though, the food you find at local farmer's markets will be organic. You do have to ask, though. Many small farmers don't use pesticides or other harmful ingredients but haven't been able to afford the organic certification process.

There are a few key ways to follow the hundred-mile rule. Find out where your nearest farmer's market is and shop there. Or join a CSA (community supported agriculture) program—local farms that let you buy a "share" of the farm or pay a monthly fee in exchange for monthly produce deliveries, often straight to your doorstep. Another option is to join a food cooperative, a member-owned business that provides groceries and other products to its members at a discount. Most of the products are organic and come from local family farms. All you do is sign up and pay some dues.

The best way to find these programs is to check the websites of government and nonprofit organizations, such as the Alternative Farming Systems Information Center (afsic.nal.usda.gov); FoodRoutes (www.foodroutes.org); Cooperative Grocers' Information Network (www.cgin.coop); and LocalHarvest (www.local harvest.org). All the info you need will pop up on your screen.

BE SEASONAL • 1 POINT

Buy and consume fruits and vegetables that are in season. It saves you money: growing foods out of season is costly. It's expensive to bend the laws of Mother Nature, and that cost is passed on to the consumer—you. Foods that are grown out of season are often sprayed with all sorts of chemicals (which make us fat) because they require artificial help to survive the strange weather in which they're brought into the world.

Seasonal foods have more nutrients, which translates into better health and a stronger metabolism, giving you an added edge when it comes to weight management. Researchers in Japan found threefold differences in the vitamin C content of spinach harvested in summer versus winter, and vitamin C is a key nutrient in combating stress and in inhibiting the fat-storage hormone cortisol.

In different parts of the world, and even in different regions of one country, seasonal options can vary. But here are some simple guidelines to help you put this tip into practice and ensure optimal nourishment:

- SPRING—Focus on leafy, dark greens like Swiss chard, spinach, romaine lettuce, fresh parsley, and basil. Asparagus and artichokes are at their peak then, too, along with fruits such as apricots, strawberries, and citrus.
- SUMMER—Center your meals on vegetables like summer squashes, tomatoes, eggplant, and corn; use herbs like mint, basil, and cilantro. Stick with light, cooling fruits like blueberries, blackberries, raspberries, boysenberries, as well as grapes, melons, sweet peaches, and plums.
- FALL—Turn toward the more warming harvest foods, including carrots, sweet potatoes, pumpkin, broccoli, cauliflower, kale, onions, and garlic. Emphasize the more warming spices and seasonings, including ginger, peppercorns, and mustard seeds. Enjoy apples and pears as they're crisp and juicy now.
- WINTER—Lean more toward root vegetables like carrots, potatoes, onions, and garlic as well as winter squashes. Citrus fruits such as mandarin oranges and clementines are plentiful, as are cranberries and pomegranates.

Whatever the season, be creative. Let the natural energy and aesthetic beauty of spring, summer, fall, and winter be your culinary inspiration.

MANAGE YOUR MEALS

DON'T SKIP • • • 3 POINTS

Don't skip any meals, especially breakfast. When you skip meals, it throws off your blood sugar and triggers insulin instability, which then causes you to overeat when you finally do eat. Studies have shown that food tastes up to 25 percent better when we are overly hungry, which naturally leads to overeating. In addition, being super-hungry depletes your willpower. How many times have you grabbed a scoop of the M&M's out of your coworker's candy bowl because you skipped breakfast or lunch and were "starving" (as well as cranky and shaky—symptoms that your blood sugar has dropped)?

Skipping meals may wreak havoc on your health as well. Researchers compared subjects who ate three meals per day versus those who had one large evening meal. They found that meal skippers showed elevated fasting glucose levels and a delayed insulin response, both possible precursors to diabetes if the habit is maintained over the long term. Skipping meals affects your ability to focus, concentrate, make decisions, and even exercise effectively. Deprive your brain too long of nutrition, and it may undergo glucose deprivation. Some sure signs that you need to eat *right now*: dizziness, confusion, sleepiness, weakness, or anxiety.

Skipping meals is a stupid mistake that there's just no excuse for. Eat something substantive within an hour of waking. Don't let more than four hours pass between meals (more on that in a moment). I don't care how busy you are—it isn't that hard to carry snacks with you, or have grab-and-go foods at the ready to avoid this diet snafu.

FOLLOW THE FOUR-BY-FOUR RULE •• 2 POINTS

Let's get some solid clarification on the timing of your meals. Not only do I not want you skipping meals, I also don't want you "grazing" throughout the day. I don't want you "eating small meals"—you know, the six-small-meals-to-boost-metabolism theory. I think that's utter crap. When you snack throughout the day or eat many small meals, you release insulin. This insulin release promotes fat storage, because your body is trying to burn off and utilize a constant flow of sugar to the bloodstream from nonstop eating.

Also, we often don't remember to count the small snacks we grab when considering our daily calorie allowance. Studies show that many people don't feel satiated from a small meal, either, which can

SLIM MYTH:

Eating small, frequent meals boosts your metabolism.

FAST FACT: This myth is based on the theory that if you keep adding small amounts of food to your fire (the fire being your metabolism), you'll keep it going strong and burn more calories overall. The exact *opposite* is true. If you keep adding food to the fire, you'll never dig into your fat stores. You're constantly releasing insulin, which puts your body in a constant "absorptive phase." In this phase, insulin not only stimulates the enzymes that help store sugar and build up fat; it also *inhibits* other enzymes that tend to release sugar from storage and break down fat. Being in a constant absorptive phase never allows your body the chance to experience the peaks and valleys of insulin and many other hormones that help balance our use of energy. (Remember, fat is stored energy.) The goal is to eat every four hours so you successfully move from the absorptive phase to the "postabsorptive phase" when your body goes into your energy stores for sustenance.

In addition, from a behavioral perspective, grazing can cause you to lose track of how much you've eaten and accidentally overeat. And psychologically it can leave you feeling unsatisfied because you never sit down and have a full meal. Follow the four-by-four rule, and it will all work out to your slim satisfaction.

then cause them to overeat throughout the day to make up for that lack of satisfaction.

I want you to eat every four hours. There's only one time of day when I want you to snack, and that's between lunch and dinner. Your snack should be something substantive. Eating every four hours stabilizes your blood sugar, optimizes insulin production, and manages hunger—all of which are critical to weight loss and weight management.

SNACK SMART •• 2 POINTS

As I mentioned in discussing the four-by-four rule, I want you to think of your snack more as a fourth meal rather than as an all-day grazing marathon. Here's how to do it right:

- Make your snack roughly 20 percent of your calorie allowance. For example, if you're eating 1,200 calories a day, then you have a 200-to-240-calorie snack.
- Make your snack a balance of macronutrients, just as you do with your meals. Eat a mix of healthy proteins, fats, and carbs.

Here are some stellar and satisfying snack examples. (Calorie counts are approximate, and may vary with brand and size.)

- 1 small apple and 7 walnuts (236 calories)
- 1 tablespoon peanut butter on 5 to 7 (depending on size) whole-grain crackers (200–215 calories)
- 1 cup sliced veggies dipped in ¼ cup hummus (224 calories)
- ⅛ cup air-popped popcorn sprinkled with 1 teaspoon shredded Parmesan cheese (240 calories)
- 6 or 7 pita chips with 2 tablespoons of black bean dip and 2 tablespoons of sliced avocado (213 calories)
- ½ cup low-fat, 2 percent cottage cheese with ½ cup fresh fruit and 10 raw almonds (222 calories)
- a 12-ounce fruit smoothie made with low-fat yogurt or milk (200 calories)
- 1 hard-boiled egg with 1 large pear (211 calories)
- 4 long celery stalks with 2 tablespoons of almond butter (224 calories)

MAKE IT A PRODUCTION •• 2 POINTS

Sit down and eat a real meal. I don't *ever* want you to eat while sitting in front of the TV or computer, standing over the sink, walking in between meetings, or riding on the subway. Even with your afternoon snack, sit down and "make a meal of it." Here's why: multitasking while you eat can make you eat more. We get caught up in mindless munching because our mind is preoccupied with something else. This can inhibit your body from sending and receiving the "I'm full!" signals that help regulate food intake. In addition, studies show that from a psychological perspective, when we don't sit down to eat, we don't fully recognize that we've eaten. As a result, we don't feel satisfied.

Research has shown that most of the foods we eat standing up are low in nutritional value and high in empty calories. A study published in the *Journal of the American Dietetic Association* demonstrated that young adults who eat on the run consume more fast foods and soft drinks, and less healthy food, than their peers who make time to sit down to dinner.

Bottom line: sit your butt down and eat with no distractions, except for the company of friends and family who can add to the enjoyment of your meal.

FOLLOW THE 80/20 RULE •• 2 POINTS

This is a fairly common bit of advice that I live by: eat great food for 80 percent of your daily calorie allowance and make 20 percent of it treat foods. So for example, if I'm eating 1,800 calories a day (remember, I'm not trying to lose weight, just maintain my weight), around 1,450 of my entire daily calories will be superhealthy stuff like fish, greens, whole grains, and so on, while 350 calories will be a cookie or a scoop of ice cream.

Every day, if I choose, I get to enjoy the things I really don't want to go without. Another good way to implement this advice is to practice meal rotation. After you eat a "cheat meal" or treat, follow it with at least five healthy meals (including snacks). Although you won't get a treat in every day, this method allows you more treat calories when you do indulge, and it still assures that you'll be eating right at least 80 percent of the time.

EZ CALORIE CUT

For 1 cup of regular ice cream, substitute 1 cup of low-fat frozen yogurt. **CUT: 121 CALORIES**

This strategy works because it keeps you from feeling deprived. Willpower will take us only so far, and when we deprive ourselves of the things we really like to eat, the desire for what we can't have can ultimately, in a "weak moment" (rough day at the office, kids driving you crazy, traffic jam—you name it), lead to a binge. Deprivation is miserable and isn't sustainable. You're not going to go the rest of your life without a bite of chocolate or a piece of pizza.

I still want you to choose the chemical-free versions of your favorite treats, though. For example, I choose Unreal brand peanut butter cups because they have no HFCS, trans fats, or other crap. Or I have Newman's Own cookies, again because they have no chemicals or junk in them.

Other people might suggest a cheat day to you instead of the 80/20 rule. I strongly recommend against it. From a psychological perspective, it has you living all week in anticipation of a binge— not good. In addition, a cheat day often has no caloric parameters built into it. Many people overconsume on their cheat day and wipe out all the hard work they put in during the week. I've seen the cheat day freak many people out, too, because they feel guilty for "going crazy" with their food. The 80/20 rule for daily eating is the way to go for weight loss and weight management. It's sustainable over the long run and effective on the scale.

BEVERAGE BASICS

DON'T DRINK YOUR CALORIES • • 2 POINTS

Most caloric drinks—like sodas and juices—are loaded with sugar and send your insulin levels skyrocketing. Plus, they don't have fiber to help you feel full, so you've just drunk 100-plus calories of liquid sugar, yet, adding insult to injury, you're still going to feel hungry.

Juice too has a ton of sugar and calories—almost as much as soda. You're much better off eating the fruit.

If you think you're going to consume the sugar-free version of these drinks to get around the calorie and sugar problem, remember my earlier tip about why we don't consume chemicals. They make us fat.

Here are some simple beverage suggestions that will quench your thirst without sinking the scale:

YES

Water, tea, and coffee (in moderation—2 strong cups a day, max) are good choices. If you find a drink that's sweetened with a natural, low-calorie sweetener like stevia or xylitol, that's okay—these sugar substitutes are not believed to cause an insulin spike. But water is always a better choice. Organic dairy or other forms of milk, like almond or coconut, are okay if you include them as part of a meal and account for them in your total daily calorie intake.

NO

Soda, juice, sugary teas, sugary flavored waters, diet drinks with artificial sweeteners, and alcohol. (For those who can't imagine following this tip, see the "two-drink maximum" tip, next.)

KEEP TO A TWO-DRINK MAXIMUM • 1 POINT

Booze makes you fat. It's very high in empty calories, and except for red wine and beer, it has little or no nutrient content. Alcohol also destroys willpower, often leading you to overeat. Worse, studies have shown that alcohol suppresses fat metabolism by as much as 70 percent. It contributes to unwanted fat storage, too, because when you drink alcohol, it's broken down into something called acetate, which your body will burn before anything else. All other extra calories will be stored as fat.

Now, I know you aren't going to give up booze entirely, so let's talk about how to do it intelligently and successfully. The first rule of thumb is to limit your intake to two drinks a week. Pick a night, make it your wild one, and have up to two drinks. If you're thinking you won't "catch a buzz," you're wrong. The less you drink, the lower your tolerance. When you don't drink much or often, two drinks should do the job.

When you do drink, choose the following:

- **Red wine.** Red wine is moderate on the calorie scale and loaded with antioxidants and health benefits. For example, the resveratrol in red wine can help prevent damage to blood vessels, reduce "bad" cholesterol, and inhibit blood clots.
- **Dark beer.** Moderate on the calorie scale and loaded with antioxidants and flavonoids, this beverage is also good for heart health.
- **Clear alcohol.** These liquors must be consumed straight, on the rocks, or with calorie-free mixers, like tequila on the rocks with a splash of lime or vodka and soda water.

If you're thinking the above recommendations are no fun and you want your Sunday-morning Bloody Mary or your Friday-night margarita, think about how fun fat is. It's not. You really get into trouble with alcohol when you start adding the sugar-laden mixers to the booze. Plus, habitual indulgence in alcohol is linked to all kinds of health-related issues, from cancer to dementia. Also, not fun. Ultimately. I want you to be grateful that I'm letting you have two drinks a week, even if they aren't fun ones, but I'm not a *total* bitch. Here are a few slimmed-down versions of common cocktails, in case you just can't live without one:

SLIM COLADA (160 CALORIES)

2 ounces SKYY Infusions Coconut

2 ounces club soda

Splash of pineapple juice

Squeeze of lemon

Mix all ingredients with ice, and serve in a highball glass.

SLIMMOJITO (140 CALORIES)

2 ounces white rum

12 mint leaves muddled in a glass

1 teaspoon Truvia sweetener

1 ounce fresh lime juice

3 ounces club soda

Mix all ingredients with ice, and serve in a highball glass.

SLIMMERITA (150 CALORIES)

1½ ounces 100% Agave Tequila Milagro Silver

½ ounce Patron Citronge Orange Liqueur (or substitute
   pomegranate juice)

4–5 ounces sparkling natural lemon- or lime-flavored mineral
   water (Trader Joe's has a good one)

Squeeze of lime

Mix all ingredients with ice, and serve in a tall glass.

FILL 'ER UP • • • 3 POINTS

We all know that water is good for weight loss; it helps curb hunger, flushes out toxins that make us sick and fat, boosts energy, and speeds metabolism by up to 3 percent. While 3 percent may not seem like a lot, when you add it up over the course of a lifetime, it makes a big difference on your waistline. I guarantee it.

There has been a lot of confusion over the years about how much water we should drink. Eight ounces a day, a cup every hour, six cups a day—the list goes on and on.

Here's the deal: our water and hydration needs vary and depend on a host of factors, which range from weather changes to activity level to our unique biochemistry. The best rule of thumb to stay optimally hydrated is to drink until your pee looks like lemonade. If it's darker in color—apple juice—you need more water. If you're taking supplements, it may be bright, and that's okay; but if it turns brownish, you need more water. It really is that simple.

If you're wondering or worrying about what type of water you should drink—as in alkaline (water that has a low pH balance) or ionized (water with ionized minerals that have an electric charge)—don't. This isn't one you need to overthink. While some research does say that alkaline and/or ionized water may be best for you, you don't need to get fancy with your water to get its slimming or health benefits. If you don't have access to these waters, or if they're too expensive, don't sweat it!

TAP IT—BOTTLED VERSUS TAP WATER • 1 POINT

What about bottled or tap? Easy! Tap. Just because water is bottled doesn't mean it's contaminant-free. In fact, it can be quite the opposite. City water is highly regulated and monitored for safety. Bottled water is not. Technically, the FDA monitors bottled water, but it turns out that about 70 percent of bottled water sold in a state is exempt from federal regulation. Many bottled waters have tested positive for bacteria, man-made chemicals, and arsenic. Going with tap saves you money and saves the environment. You keep the landfills from overflowing with plastic bottles and you reduce carbon emissions caused by transporting the water from distant locations to your fridge.

But wait—you're not out of the woods yet. Drinking tap water still leaves you at risk for lead, chlorine, pesticides, fungicides, herbicides, hormones, antibiotics, and nitrates. You can check on the quality of your local water by calling the EPA's safe water hotline at (800) 426-4791 or check out its website: www.epa.gov/safewater.

Your best bet is to filter your tap water. Reverse osmosis filters are a great option. They remove all heavy metals and viruses and some pharmaceuticals. Or you can go with an activated carbon filter like Brita. The quality varies from product to product, but most will remove heavy metals, pesticides, and some pharmaceuticals.

Last thought on water: bubbly versus flat? Carbonated water is created (or exists naturally) by dissolving carbon dioxide (CO_2) in water. This creates carbonic acid, which is more acidic than regular water (it falls somewhere in the range of apple and orange juice) but is much less acidic than your stomach. It's important to understand that the human body maintains pH equilibrium on a constant basis and that its pH will not be affected by water consumption. Some concern exists regarding tooth enamel erosion due to the increased acidity, but a 2001 study in the *Journal of Oral Rehabilitation* showed that while sparkling mineral waters showed slightly greater erosive potential than still waters, the potential was considered low and was on the order of one hundred times less than that of soft drinks.

Some bottled or canned carbonated water contains added sodium to decrease the acidity and improve taste. If you're on a low-sodium diet and consume bottled or canned carbonated water, make sure to pay attention to the sodium content and choose lower-sodium options.

When all is said and done, hydration is the most important part of this equation. Just drink water, carbonated or flat, alkaline, ionized, or plain—until you pee lemonade.

SLIM MYTH:

I can slim down by switching to diet soda.

FAST FACT: Chuggin' that crap is definitely pudging up your paunch. Remember our conversation about chemical obesogens? A study at Purdue University found that rats given artificial sweeteners ate more calories and gained more weight than rats given sugar. Stick with water!

USE FLAVORFUL DISGUISES • 1 POINT

All right, if you've decided to turn in your soda can for a glass of water—but you simply cannot stomach the thought of drinking it plain—here's a great tip for you. Flavor your water with cranberry, pomegranate, apple, lime, or grape juice—add just a splash to banish the bland. Be sure to choose all-natural, pure juice, not the cocktail versions with tons of added sugar and crap.

A product I love called Soda Stream allows you to create your own natural sodas. You can customize the carbonation of your water (lightly fizzy, medium, or super bubbly) and add whatever natural juice you like most. It's great for the environment, saves you a fortune, is good for getting your water quota in, and is a godsend for those struggling to give up sodas. Bob Harper and I swear by this machine; it helped us both tremendously when we wanted to kick our diet soda habits once and for all.

DO SMALL, NOT TALL • 1 POINT

If you're one of those professed nonwater drinkers, try using a small glass (highball or juice) and drinking it all in one swoop. That's one down—only a few more to go. You can easily repeat it throughout the day. By evening, you'll be surprised how much water you drank with ease and without the angst of staring at a tall, full bottle throughout the day.

EAT WATER-PACKED FOODS • 1 POINT

If you tend to not drink enough water *and* you're a nosher, include foods in your diet that have naturally high water content and low calorie counts, such as watermelon, zucchini, and cucumbers. These can add water to your daily intake and let you munch without eating up your calorie allowance—literally.

ADD IT UP, DROP IT OFF

GIVE YOURSELF 3 POINTS

- [ ] Live in the red.
- [ ] Get the lowdown.
- [ ] Clear out the kitchen cabinets.
- [ ] Downsize: switch to "slim-size" portions.
- [ ] Discriminate—don't eliminate.
- [ ] Don't eat chemical crap.
- [ ] Don't skip.
- [ ] Fill 'er up.

GIVE YOURSELF 2 POINTS

- [ ] Write it down, add it up.
- [ ] Bag it.
- [ ] Baby-step your way to fewer calories.
- [ ] Land, sea, or tree.
- [ ] Go back to nature.
- [ ] Keep it clean.
- [ ] Forget about fat-free.
- [ ] Eat in Technicolor.
- [ ] Follow the four-by-four rule.
- [ ] Snack smart.
- [ ] Make it a production.
- [ ] Follow the 80/20 rule.
- [ ] Don't drink your calories.

GIVE YOURSELF 1 POINT

- [ ] Go local.
- [ ] Be seasonal.
- [ ] Keep to a two-drink maximum.
- [ ] Tap it—bottled versus tap water.
- [ ] Use flavorful disguises.
- [ ] Do small, not tall.
- [ ] Eat water-packed foods.

_____ Total *points* for Chapter 1

_____ Total number of *tips* I'm incorporating

CHAPTER 2

MOVING

As I mentioned in Chapter 1's "Live in the red" tip, you have to burn roughly 3,500 calories to lose a pound. (Your personal number could be higher or lower.) While most likely you'll have to eat less to achieve this deficit, the true speed of your results, and the maintenance as well, will be highly dependent upon the how, when, and why of your exercise regimen. Following a healthy diet is imperative to keep you from gaining weight, but to truly shed the pounds and shred your physique, a smart, powerful fitness regimen is equally important.

The following tips and tricks are perhaps some of the most important in this book. You have to move to lose weight and/or to maintain a sexy slim physique, *but* you don't have to work out for hours and hours to get amazing results. Just as with your food choices, the key is the *quality* of your training, not necessarily the quantity. So pay close attention, because what you're about to learn is going to save you hours and hours of time, blow your mind, transform your body, and make your workouts way more manageable and enjoyable.

....

Cracking the Exercise Code

THE FOUNDATION

DRESS FOR THE PART • 1 POINT

Proper gear is key to both safety and performance. Wear comfortable, properly fitted footwear and clothing that's appropriate to the weather and the activity. It's worth the initial investment, trust me. I remember when I first got into road biking, I thought the whole getup looked ridiculous. The pants with the butt pad made me feel like I was wearing a diaper. So I went on a ride one day in my sweats. By the end of it, I thought the seat was going to have to be surgically removed from my backside. Take it from me—having the right gear is critical.

If you don't know what to buy, ask someone who is well versed in the sport. My horse trainer helped me buy the proper boots for my height and level of skill. My surf instructor made sure I bought the proper wetsuit for my size, gender, and the water temperature I usually surf in. A great place to start is to go to a shoe store or a sporting goods store and ask the salesperson. Different sports require different features and functions in their attire, so make sure you specify what you'll be doing. Have the salesperson help you take into account your anatomy, gait, level of fitness, and so on, based on your sport or activity.

As a rule of thumb, buy your shoes a half-size larger than you normally wear, as feet tend to swell during exercise. You can get by with a great pair of cross trainers; they're constructed for heavy usage. If you're pursuing a specific sport or activity and are really focused on it, it's better if you purchase shoes to optimize both comfort and performance. If you want to run, then get running shoes. And don't wear them for your cardio classes at the gym—they don't provide enough lateral support. Same goes for indoor cycling, CrossFit, or dance, whatever your sport.

When it comes to what to wear, you want to wear clothing that doesn't restrict your movement. You'll want tops, pants, and socks made of wicking fabrics, which have special properties to draw the moisture away from your skin and back into the fabric, so you and your clothes don't end up being a sweaty mess. Fabrics like organic cotton, merino wool, and bamboo, to name a few, offer a multitude of benefits that can enhance the workout experience and are absolutely worth the investment. Look for clothes with fabrics that have:

- Thermal control—temperature-regulating properties to keep you warm in cold weather and cool when it's hot
- UPF—ultraviolet protection against harmful sun rays, fused right into the fabric
- Compression—special Lycra or elastic-type fibers that hold you in tight or have specially placed panels to remind you to, well, suck it in
- Antibacterial and antimicrobrial properties—these translate to odor-free!
- Insect repellent—if you're outdoors and in a tropical climate, these are a must. You won't smell a thing, but the fabric will keep the mosquitoes and other nasty bugs away.

If you want to feel and perform like a lean, mean, rockin' fitness machine, gear up for it. If you feel great about how you look, chances are you'll train a little harder and be more enthused to hit the gym.

CONSISTENCY IS KEY • • • 3 POINTS

For years I told people that the best time of day to work out was whenever they could manage to fit it into their schedule. For some, that meant first thing in the morning; for others, it meant after work or at night, once things settled down for the day. Now, however, new research suggests that the answer is to be found in *consistency*. The best time to work out is the same time every day. Your body gets conditioned to exercise at this time and adapts to it by releasing energy boosting, muscle-building hormones like testosterone that aid in fitness performance and fat metabolism. If you can get into a consistent routine, you might eke out a little extra oomph in your performance, which in turn burns more calories. If not, don't stress it—the most important thing is that you work out regularly (4 to 6 times a week), no matter the time of day.

DO A FIVE-MINUTE WARM-UP
• 1 POINT

A study in the *Journal of Applied Physiology* found that lengthy warm-ups can fatigue you, particularly if you're warming up with static, held stretches. According to numerous studies, improper warm-ups actually put your muscles in sleep mode. That's no good; you want your muscles ready for action! Five minutes of cardio and/or dynamic stretches (active stretching with fluid movement, as opposed to a static stretch like the sit-and-reach toe touch) will get the job done and have you ready to up the ante for the main part of the workout. Any form of cardio will do, as long as it gets your heart rate up and literally warms up your body, even breaking you into a light sweat. Try the bike, treadmill, or rowing

---

SLIM MYTH:

Static stretching before working out is crucial to preventing injury.

FAST FACT: Static stretching after a workout can be beneficial, but static stretching before a workout doesn't increase your range of motion. Some studies suggest that stretching may actually destabilize muscles and weaken them by up to 30 percent, making them less prepared for strenuous exercise, especially if you're doing something like weight lifting. So stick to warming up with dynamic, active movements like arm and leg swings, simple squats, easy jogging, or even a march—you'll be better prepared for whatever your activity and run less risk.

machine; you can even jump rope or use old-school calisthenics like jumping jacks. As for the active stretches, try movements like toe taps (hold your arms out at your sides, hinge at the hips, drop down and diagonally touch your left arm to your right foot and repeat on the other side), arm circles, hip circles, torso twists, lunges, easy squats, or even cat and cow poses from yoga class.

The takeaway here: yes, you need to warm up for the hard stuff. Don't just jump right in. Your body needs a gradual rise in heart rate, joint lubrication, and mental prep. But when done right, you should only need and take 5 minutes to do it.

REMODEL YOUR MUSCLES • • • 3 POINTS

Can you really keep off the weight you've lost? Can you really rev your metabolism? The answer to both these questions is yes and yes. The key to doing it is that you have to lift (as in weight training) to lose. If you've got pounds to peel off, strength training is your E-ticket: *E* as in "energy utilized." Let me explain. How many times have you heard that if you had more muscle, more lean tissue, it would increase your fat-burning, calorie-burning capability, even while you're sleeping? Researchers have come to understand only recently the process your muscles go through after strength training. Not only does this process add muscle tissue; in the *afterburn, your muscles are being remodeled.*

I always tell you to push and work to true fatigue, and here's why: when you do, your muscles go through a normal rebuilding process. This occurs naturally with any strength training. This remodeling process takes 24 to 96 hours to complete after you've trained (which is another reason why you must build rest into your weekly routine). During this time, satellite cells surround the muscle fibers and supply protein to them so that new muscle tissue develops with higher strength capabilities. What creates the additional calorie burn, to the tune of 100 to 105 calories per day, is the afterburn energy used for the remodeling.

Regular weight training results in a real increase in your resting metabolic rate that you can count on—as long as you keep training. Let me give you some calorie-burning perspective: 30 minutes of steady-state cardio will burn about 300 calories. But unlike the case with strength training, no remodeling process follows cardio work, so there's a minimal afterburn. In a 30-minute resistance workout, you'll burn around the same 300 calories. The difference is that you'll burn an additional 100 calories per day for three days after your workout! Which would you rather do: burn 300 calories for cardio or 600 calories for one resistance training session? One strength-training workout per week can help you burn 31,000 to 36,000 extra calories or 9 to 10 pounds of fat in one year! Now you know—I want you doing strength training at least twice a week so these numbers can double.

If you want to lose weight, speed up your metabolism, and burn more calories, do your strength training in circuits, as mentioned in the next paragraph. This type of training is called metabolic resistance training (MRT), sometimes referred to as metabolic circuit training (MCT) because, in effect, you're heavily (no pun intended) influencing your metabolism.

STAY IN MOTION • • • 3 POINTS

There are many different ways to approach your workout. But when it comes to weight loss in *Slim for Life*, there is one method that will rip weight off your body as fast as possible: circuit training. Circuit training is when you do sets of strength and/or conditioning exercises back to back, one right after the other, with little or no rest in between moves. This type of training provides the best of both cardio and strength in one workout because it trains and tones the muscles while simultaneously challenging the cardiovascular system. It saves time and maximizes your calorie burn, because there's never a wasted moment.

With this kind of efficiency, you don't have to spend crazy-long hours exercising, which leaves more time for some of those other things you might want to do. All my workout programs—from my BODYSHRED class to my DVDs to my book *Making the Cut*—were all created using exercise circuits. Here's an example of a good basic circuit using familiar exercises to do after you warm up:

CIRCUIT 1

Push-ups

Squats with a Dumbbell Shoulder Press

Bench Triceps Dips

Jumping Jacks

You essentially move from one exercise to the next with no break in between, performing each exercise for a full 30 seconds. Upon completion of the circuit, you can take a brief 30-second rest, then repeat the entire group of exercises for a second circuit. For exercises that require external weight like a dumbbell, use enough weight to fatigue the muscle you're working by the end of that time, which I prefer to counting reps.

This discussion might also answer any questions you have about whether to do cardio or focus on strength. I want you to do pure cardio only on the days you aren't doing your circuit training, as it's far less efficient than circuits.

Why not do circuit training every day if it gets a much better burn during and after the workout? This is a no-no—check out what's next, to understand why.

SPLIT IT UP AND TAKE A LOAD OFF •• 2 POINTS

Many fitness enthusiasts spend a lot of time training but very little time acknowledging the power and necessity of recovery. In fact, most of your gains are going to be made on your recovery days.

Exercise is the architect, but recovery is the builder. Without properly timed recovery, you'll stress your body, inhibit your progress, and possibly injure yourself.

What should you do instead? Make sure you take at least one day completely off each week from exercise. Don't train a muscle group *intensely* more than twice a week. And most researchers agree that you should make sure to allow 48 to 72 hours of rest in between exercise sessions, particularly the more intense ones where you're doing heavy resistance training,

How do you do this and still move 5 to 6 days a week, which I recommend? Don't worry, I'm about to show you. We utilize a technique called muscle splits. You create your circuits to work certain muscle groups on certain days, but not all muscle groups on the same day. If you're confused, don't be. I'll illustrate the ideal muscle split and workout schedule for you below. But before I do, I want to clarify something: full-body training, where you hit every muscle group in the same workout, can produce some amazing results. It just doesn't allow you to optimize recovery time, so you either can't do it every day, or you can't work out as intensely.

In my perfect world, though, you can exercise in a hard-core way five to six days a week and still get your needed recovery for your muscles and subsequently ramp up your results.

Your training "splits" (muscles you train on the same day) would look as follows:

Day 1: Chest, Triceps, Shoulders, Legs with Quadricep Focus, Lower-fiber Abs, Obliques

Day 2: Back, Biceps, Legs with Hamstring Focus, Glutes, Upper-fiber Abs

Day 3: Cardio

Day 4: Chest, Triceps, Shoulders, Legs with Quadricep Focus, Lower-fiber Abs, Obliques

Day 5: Back, Biceps, Legs with Hamstring Focus, Glutes, Upper-
    fiber Abs
Day 6: Cardio
Day 7: Day Off

I paired these muscle groups together for a reason based on function. Chest, shoulders, triceps, and quadriceps are all push muscles,
while back, biceps, and hamstrings are pull muscles; hamstrings and
glutes generally work in tandem, so it's a pairing that makes training sense. Muscles with the same function generally work together
to perform an exercise, so it's ideal to train them on the same day. If
you don't train muscles with the same function on the same days, it
would be nearly impossible to maximize your strength during workouts and your recovery afterward. For example, if you do biceps
curls on Monday, but then you do lat rows (which recruits biceps as
assisting muscles) on Tuesday, you'll be working biceps two days in
a row whether you realize it or not. In addition, your back workout
will suffer because the biceps will be too fatigued from the workout
the day before.

On split days, I like to incorporate a technique called Peripheral
Heart Action (PHA). PHA training typically alternates upper-body
and lower-body moves, in order to give the muscle just worked a
break without letting the body rest or the burn slow down. Circuit training, which you already will be doing, tends to be PHA by
design—another reason it's so effective. This technique forces
blood flow to continuously circulate throughout the whole body by
repeatedly changing muscle groups as well as muscle destination
(upper to lower or vice versa), which drives heart rate and acceler-
ates calorie burn. The key is to put the emphasis on large muscle
groups like chest, back, and legs, which require a higher cardio out-
put demand on the heart, resulting in a more metabolically driven
workout.

Here's a sample PHA circuit for both muscle split days:

MONDAY AND THURSDAY
Dumbbell Chest Presses on a Stability Ball

Squats with Anterior Front Raises

Triceps Dips, on the floor or using a bench

High Knees (HIIT INTERVAL, see page 54, "Push it good," for more)

Leg Raises, either alternate (easier version) or both legs

TUESDAY AND FRIDAY
Lat Pull-downs or Bent-over High Rows with Dumbbells

Straight-Leg Dead Lifts into Biceps Curls

Seated Lat Rows

Butt Kicks (HIIT INTERVAL)

Crunches on a Stability Ball

Now, if you're working classes into your schedule, think about what muscles they train. Suppose you do yoga on Monday: by nature of the exercises—lots of planks, chatarungas, and downward-facing dogs—it's very chest, shoulders, and triceps intensive. So don't take a boot camp class on Tuesday, where push-ups, presses, and dips will be used on these same muscle groups—they are prime exercises in most boot camps. Instead, take the class that targets more of the lower body, like a Below the Belt Butt Blaster. While this might take slightly more planning on your part, I assure you it's worth the effort and will make an enormous difference in the speed of your results.

If you're doing a workout DVD or a class where you train your total body, that's okay—as long as the workout doesn't overly focus on a certain muscle group and is more focused on overall conditioning and burning calories. My BODYSHRED class, for example, is only

30 minutes long and it touches on every muscle in the body, but it doesn't hammer one muscle group in particular.

Ultimately, I don't want you to strength-train a muscle if it's still sore from a previous workout. That's the golden rule. And to reiterate, make sure to take at least one full day off from exercise a week for optimal recovery and results.

PUT IT TOGETHER • • • 3 POINTS

When you're doing your strength training, I want you to think about efficiency. I pair small muscles together with big muscles in the same exercise because synergizing multiple muscle groups simultaneously requires a tremendous amount of energy and produces a higher calorie burn. Working smaller muscle groups like biceps, shoulders, or triceps, along with legs, makes substantially better use of your time. This is essentially what you're doing in the split circuits I just discussed.

There are several ways to do this, and I define these types of moves in three ways: Combo Lifts, Mash Ups, and Shredders. A Combo Lift is when you perform one exercise, then directly move into another without resting. A Mash Up is when you perform two moves at the same time. A Shredder is a move that organically trains multiple muscle groups at the same time and has you moving and changing position. Combo Lifts are easier because they don't require as much coordination, strength, or stability as a Mash Up or a Shredder, so start with these and work your way up. Here are some sample moves for you to try:

> **SLIM MYTH:**
>
> **Crunches and ab workouts will get rid of belly fat.**
>
> **FAST FACT:** You can't spot-reduce fat. Not on your abs, buns, thighs, or any other place on your physique that you seek to transform. To tone up your problem areas, you have to first reduce your overall body fat, which means high-intensity training combined with clean eating and spot-specific exercises to condition the muscle under the fat.

COMBO LIFTS

Squat into an Overhead Shoulder Press

Sumo Squat into an Overhead Triceps Extension

Dead Lift into a Wide Upright Row

Forward Lunge into Biceps Curls

Curtsy Lunge into a Lateral Raise

MASH UPS

Side Lunge with Posterior Shoulder Raise

Plank with Alternating Dumbbell Row

Rear Lunge with Hammer Biceps Curls

Forward Lunge with Dumbbell Chop

Side Squat with Scooping Dumbbell Chest Fly

SHREDDERS

You may have noticed the exercises I've listed in this chapter are fairly self-explanatory or easily looked up for the novice. With many of the Shredders, though, the name doesn't tell you all you need to know, so I've given you a brief description on how to perform it. You can also find most of these on the Internet, if you would like a visual example.

Hip Heists—From a crouch position on all fours (balls of the feet and palms on the floor), bring your right knee under and across your body toward your left armpit. Then bring your left arm back behind you so you rotate your body to face upward, knees bent, balancing on heels and palms. Then rotate back to the start position by bringing the right heel under and across your body toward your left shoulder, while bringing your left arm around and over. Then repeat on the opposite side.

Crab Walk—Sit on the floor with knees bent, arms straight, and hands placed close to the hips, fingers pointing forward. Lift into a bridge position and "walk" 4 steps forward and 4 steps back, making sure to walk the opposite foot and hand at the same time.

Bear Crawl—Get on all fours with knees lifted so they don't touch the floor, and crawl forward 4 steps, then back 4 steps. Make sure to move the opposite hand and foot simultaneously.

Rolling Side Plank Kicks—Lie sideways, propped on your forearm with your knees bent. Lift your torso up into a side plank. While balanced on the bottom knee, extend your top leg out to the side in a side-kick or locked-out position with foot flexed. Lower to the mat, roll onto your other side, and repeat the side plank and kick. Roll back. Continue to alternate sides.

Turkish Get-ups—Lie face up, one arm extended vertically, while holding a light dumbbell. Sit up, cross legs, and stand, keeping arm extended, then reverse and return to lying. Repeat, holding dumbbell with same hand for 30 seconds, then hold dumbbell in the other hand for a second pass.

The possibilities are endless, and the results are fast and furious. Plus, training in this fashion will save you time and make your body far more functional.

SECOND TIME'S A CHARM • • 2 POINTS

Often people ask me how many sets or how many reps to perform of a certain exercise. It's likely, if you've been seeking this information, that you've heard differing advice, from doing low reps with heavy weight to high reps with low weight. Or maybe you've heard to vary your sets with your reps, as in one week do one set of 50 reps then the next week do three sets of 20 reps. While there's nothing wrong with mixing things up in this way, there's an ideal number of sets for *Slim for Life* and a way to answer the reps question as well.

The key to getting results is to fatigue your muscles, so it's often recommended that you do more than one set of an exercise if not three, four, or five. My issue: I don't want you to be repetitive with your training. I would rather you train your muscles from all different angles with a variety of exercises than repeat one move for multiple sets. When you train a muscle with diversity both in exercise and angles, you hit more muscle fibers and condition the muscle more thoroughly, leading to better and faster results. (More on this in the next tip.)

The ideal is for you to perform two sets of each exercise (which should be built into a circuit format, remember?), for 30 seconds per exercise, as I said earlier, as opposed to a set number of reps. Since I'm big on no repeats with your moves to add variety and boost results, you might wonder why I don't tell you to just do one set. The answer is that if you're working unilaterally (on one side), you must repeat the set to train the other side. For example, if you do a set of pendulum lunges with biceps curls on the right leg, you obviously need to do a second set so you can train the left leg equally.

And the reason I like 30 seconds as far as reps are concerned is that that time frame allows you to max out your potential. You can still play with heavier and lighter weights, but the key is to do as many as you can in that 30 seconds with good form. Under this guideline your body will automatically adjust the reps according to capability.

ANGLE IT! •• 2 POINTS

For *Slim for Life*, I've got you doing two sets of 30 seconds each per exercise so you can optimize your workout with a variety of moves to fatigue your muscles. By training the same muscles in multiple directions or angles, you create better muscle tension and fire up more muscle fibers! Plus, it helps you avoid a training plateau, where your muscles are so accustomed to doing the same exercises in the same way that they simply cease to respond as effectively.

I'm going to get just a little science-y for a sec, but I'll try to keep it simple. Here's the deal. Take your shoulders, for example: you have muscle fibers running in three directions—front, side, and rear—which comprise the three parts of your shoulders or deltoids. If you want defined, sexy shoulders, with striated cuts that show when you lift your arm, you must hit the shoulder from all angles. If you train only with front arm raises and never lift from the side or rear, those other muscle fibers essentially don't get taxed, and there goes your shoulder definition.

So remember to use diversification with your exercises in order to hit the muscles from different angles and accelerate to insane results.

PUMP IT UP •• 2 POINTS

Forget the "target fat-burning zone"—you know, that moronic theory that during your workout you should exercise at a moderate intensity (65 to 70 percent of your maximum heart rate) to burn predominantly fat calories. That's utter crap and a massive waste of time. The exact opposite is true. For exceptional results, you want to be working out at a higher overall intensity of around 85 percent of your maximum heart rate.

Let me explain. During physical training, your body has three possible sources of energy: glucose and glycogen (blood sugar and sugar stored in the muscles), fat, and protein. Protein is a last resort—of the three energy sources, your body is least likely to draw on its protein. Whether your body takes energy from its sugar stores or its fat stores depends on the intensity of your workout. Training at a high level of intensity forces your body to draw upon a higher percentage of its glucose and glycogen stores, because they're a more efficient source of fuel, which your body will need during intense training. If you're training at low intensity, your body doesn't need to be as efficient, so it will draw on a higher percentage of fat calories for fuel.

It sounds like low-intensity training would be more effective when it comes to losing fat, right? *Wrong*. These physiological facts have led to the mistaken belief that low-intensity training is better than high-intensity training when it comes to burning fat and losing weight.

The truth is that even though a higher *percentage* of fat calories are used during low-intensity exercise, the *total* number of fat calories used during high-intensity training is greater because more overall calories are burned. Let me illustrate my point with two studies, one from the *New England Journal of Medicine* and the other from the American College of Sports Medicine (ACSM).

The first study shows that a 200-pound guy who walks 3 miles per hour on a level surface for 60 minutes burns 5.25 calories a minute. Now, when the same guy jogs at 6 miles per hour for 60 minutes, he burns 16.22 calories per minute. Okay, let's take a look at the math here. Jogging and working out at a higher intensity burned 975 calories compared to the 315 calories that he burned walking and working out a lower intensity. He burned 660 more *total calories*.

In the second study, ten subjects exercised at a low intensity, walking 3.8 miles per hour for 30 minutes. They burned 8 calories a minute, equaling 240 total calories. Of the 240 calories burned, 59 percent (144 calories) came from glucose and glycogen and 41 percent (96 calories) came from fat. This same group then exercised for 30 minutes at 6.5 miles per hour, burning 15 calories a minute. They burned 450 total calories, with 76 percent from glucose and glycogen (342 calories) and 24 percent from fat (108 calories). So they burned 210 total calories more (450–240) and 12 more fat calories, too (108–96).

As you can see, even though the percentage of fat calories burned is higher during low-intensity training, during the high-intensity workout you're burning many more fat calories and many more total calories overall.

But wait—there's more. What do you think happens to glucose

and glycogen calories that don't get burned? They turn into stored fat. That's why, at the end of the day, the main determinant of weight loss is quantity of calories burned, not the composition of the calories burned.

My last thought on this, I promise. If you exercise at a higher heart rate and intensity, your body will burn far more calories long after that workout is over. This, as I mentioned earlier, is called afterburn. One of the advantages of training at greater intensity, particularly with strength training, is that it can boost your metabolism so that you're actually burning more calories at a resting or base level. Your body becomes more efficient from training so you become a calorie-burning furnace—that's the goal!

As I mentioned, I want you working at 85 percent of your maximum heart rate while training. To figure out what this number is and how to attain it, simply plug your info into this simple equation:

Subtract your age from the number 220. This will give you your maximum heart rate (MHR). So if I am 38, my MHR is 220 − 38 = 182. Then I want to work predominantly at around 85 percent of that number, except from when I throw my HIIT (high-intensity interval training—more on that soon) Interval into the mix (which works at nearly 100 percent MHR). So I multiply 0.85 times 182 and end up with 155 beats a minute. You don't need a heart rate monitor to track this, even though it would be helpful. All you have to do is stop and count your heartbeats for six seconds during your training and then multiply by 10. I know that I need my heart to beat 15 to 16 times every six seconds to be at 155 beats a minute, working optimally at 85 percent of my MHR.

Knowing your heart rate lets you become more familiar with what intensity it takes for you to optimally burn calories. If you want an easier way to track it: you shouldn't be gasping for air while working out, but carrying on a conversation should be a struggle.

MIX IT UP •• 2 POINTS

Don't get stuck in a workout rut. Instead, mix up your workouts on a regular basis. Doing this provides multiple benefits. First, it keeps your mind from getting bored. Second, it keeps your body from plateauing for both physical performance and weight loss. Third, it's critical for your overall health as well as your fitness efficiency that you train with "holistic equality." That means you need to work your body to emphasize many different skills—speed, power, agility, balance, flexibility—to become a more well-rounded athlete. This is great for preventing injury and for enhancing your exercise capabilities—and you'll get a better calorie burn.

If you're thinking, *I don't know how to train myself in all these different ways,* the simple fix is to take a variety of classes. Most gyms, if you belong to one, have a wide range of class offerings. You can basically take a different class every day. To keep it fresh, take a yoga class for flexibility and core strength; take a boot camp class for power, speed, muscle endurance, and agility; and take an indoor cycling class for cardio stamina and leg strength. Or take a class that offers it all, like kickboxing. I endeavored to do this with BODYSHRED, and it not only gets people lean, it makes them truly fit.

I don't want you to overthink this one. Just try new things with your fitness by experimenting with different workout types. If you do so, it will all fall into place for you automatically.

MAXIMIZE YOUR MUSCLE

PUSH IT GOOD ••• 3 POINTS

Want to get slim while putting in less time at the gym? Then you need to learn to HIIT it right. HIIT stands for high-intensity interval training. If any term has been overused in fitness over the last couple of years, this may be it, but for a very good reason. HIIT is an exercise strategy that alternates periods of short, intense anaerobic exercise with less-intense recovery periods. Current research clearly shows that if you want the most efficient cardio workout, HIIT is it. If you compare high-intensity interval training with continuous, steady-state training, there really is no contest; HIIT is *the* game changer when it comes to calorie burn and fat utilization.

Numerous studies have looked at this type of intermittent training—alternating high- and low-intensity cardio, whether it's walking/running on a treadmill, cycling, or you name it—and the end results point to the same conclusion: HIIT burns more fat and creates a greater afterburn than does steady training at a lower heart rate. For those who must know, this afterburn is called excess post-exercise oxygen consumption (EPOC).

Researchers have also found that HIIT workouts seem to elevate metabolism significantly more than other forms of cardio. The last reason to do HIIT, as if these two aren't enough, is that your workouts will be significantly shorter! You don't need 60 minutes when 20 to 30 minutes of hard, busting-it-out intervals will give you more than the hour you're struggling to get through.

While HIIT sessions are traditionally short and utilize a cardio workout, I've adapted the philosophy to incorporate it into any type of workout, whether it's cardio or strength training.

During your weekly splits, you can do HIIT on your two cardio days or during circuit training. Simply work a high-intensity cardio interval into the end of your circuit for 30 seconds to a minute.

SLIM MYTH:

Always work a muscle to failure.

FAST FACT: While you may have read in some muscle magazine that pushing your body to the max during every single workout is a great idea, it's not. It can lead to overtraining, decreased strength, and potential injury. Work to the point of fatigue (the point where you could do one more rep but you'd have to cheat on form to do it) but not failure.

Researchers target 30 seconds to two minutes as the ideal window for pushing the intensity ceiling. To perform HIIT correctly, you want to target 85 to 100 percent effort, then recover. I like shorter bouts myself, because you can push the top end for a shorter time. Trust me—if you do any of the following exercises at the intensity I'm asking you to, you won't be able to continue for longer than 2 minutes; that's the beauty and the efficiency of HIIT. Don't think you can do an hour of mountain climbers and burn 900 calories in an hour; I know you're going there. These moves are meant to be intense and short, and you get this kind of calorie burn only if you're exercising at above 89 percent intensity.

Here are a few exercises to choose from:

- Switch Jump Lunges—12 calories per minute
- Squat Jumps—13 calories per minute
- Jumping Jacks—13.5 calories per minute
- Speed Skaters—13.5 calories per minute
- Mountain Climbers—15 calories per minute
- Butt Kicks—12 calories per minute
- High Knees—13 calories per minute
- Jump Rope—11 calories per minute

And here's a sample circuit. The first four exercises are resistance and conditioning moves; the last exercise is a HIIT interval:

- Assisted Pull-ups (unless of course you can do them without help) or Bent-over High Rows
- Pendulum Lunges (same leg, a front lunge followed by a rear lunge) with Corkscrew Biceps Curls (curls that rotate from palms out to palms up)
- Seated Rows
- Double Under Jump Rope (two rotations of the rope per jump)

When you're using HIIT on a cardio day, a classic example of the HIIT protocol is Tabata, with a 2-to-1 ratio, as in 20 seconds of high intensity as hard as you can go followed by a 10-second rest. You repeat this pattern for 8 intervals. Yes, it lasts only 4 minutes. That isn't sustainable for the average person but is best for advanced athletes. I've modified the principles a bit so they work better for beginning to intermediate athletes, so it's manageable yet extremely effective. Following this protocol, I can rip 500 calories off one of my *Biggest Loser* contestants in 30 minutes. So the high-to-low-intensity ratio I recommend is 30 seconds of max intensity (90 to 100 percent) followed by 30 seconds of lower intensity at roughly 50 percent effort.

Regardless of which of your workouts you work HIIT into, these short, intense routines hugely improve athletic capacity and conditioning, lead to better glucose metabolism, and dramatically enhance fat burning.

SPEED IT UP ·· 2 POINTS
You can play with the speed of your repetitions to challenge your body and increase your calorie burn. When it comes to rep speed, most people stick with the tried and true: a slow and controlled pace of about 2 seconds on the positive (lifting, pushing, or pulling the weight) and about 2 seconds on the negative (lowering or releasing the weight). This is totally fine, but if you're looking to get more out of your workout, consider lifting faster for the positive part of the repetition during a few of your weekly workouts. Superfast and explosive reps can help you build more strength and power while increasing your burn and helping to shed more fat.

On these speed reps, lift, push, or pull during the positive contraction as fast as you can with good form. (If you can't maintain good form, lessen the amount of weight you're lifting.) Then lower the weight *with control* for 2 to 4 seconds back to the start position. Don't use speed for the negative portion of the rep—*ever*!

For those of you who are wondering about negatives or slow reps for the purposes of slim, don't do them. Some studies show an increase in muscle size from this methodology, but they don't note significant changes in conditioning or fat burning. It's more effective as a bodybuilding technique for gain in muscle size. And I don't want your heart rate to drop while you're working at a decelerated pace. You don't have to speed-lift for every workout, but at least once a week be sure to change up your rep speeds, just as you change up other aspects of your workouts—to build strength and power and accelerate fat metabolism.

DOUBLE DOWN •• 2 POINTS

Meet the aptly named "superset"—a safe and natural way to get leaner and stronger in a shorter period of time. There are different types of supersets, but for our agenda, we are going to do same-muscle-group supersets. This is an advanced training method in which you do two exercises for the same muscle group, one after the other, with no rest in between. Superset training has several primary advantages over conventional, straight-set training. When supersetting, you're getting rid of the rest period between sets and adding intensity to your workouts, and as we know, more intensity means better results. Supersets allow you to overload your muscles without using heavy weights—perfect for someone who wants to get lean, and to improve their strength and endurance, without gaining size.

Here are some examples of effective supersets:

- Lat Pull-downs followed by Plank Dumbbell Rows
- Push-ups followed by Cable Chest Flys
- Leg Extensions followed by Jump Scissor Lunges

- Bicycle Crunches followed by Leg Raises
- Dead Lifts followed by Roman Chair Back Extensions
- Alternating Front Lunges followed by Jump Squats

And here's how supersetting might look in a circuit format:

- Dumbbell Chest Presses
- Dumbbell Chest Flys with Pelvic Thrusts
- Supermans
- Mountain Climbers

GIVE YOURSELF LEVERAGE •• 2 POINTS

Your muscles, bones, and joints act as a system of levers that work together and allow you to lift weight, whether it's your own body weight or external resistance like a dumbbell. As you increase the distance between the object you're lifting and the joint (the pivot point) that's moving, your muscles must generate more force. Essentially, by extending the length of the lever—your arms, legs, or torso—you put your muscles at a disadvantage. They have to use more force to do the same job, making you stronger and leaner at the same time. Here's an example of what I mean: when you're doing push-ups on your hands and feet, then drop to your knees, you have essentially shortened the lever, and it's far easier. Our goal is to make it harder, so we burn more and get better results faster. We want to make the levers longer when we train.

Here are some ways to apply this technique:

- Do push-ups on your hands and feet—even if your hands are on an elevated platform like a step.
- Do lateral raises with straight arms instead of bent ones.
- Do dumbbell flys or cable flys instead of using a pec deck machine, where arms are bent.

- If you do leg raises, straighten your leg instead of bending it at the knee.

If you're still confused as to how best to perform an exercise to maximum effectiveness, follow this guideline: keep your body as long as possible at all times. If you have an option to perform a move with bent legs or straight legs, or with bent arms or straight arms, choose straight for a more intense workout.

Here's the caveat for all: do the harder version only as long as you can maintain perfect form. You may have to build up to it. I'd rather you try a few harder ones, and then do the easier versions perfectly, than never try. You'll build strength and amp up results by continually adding more of the challenging versions to your workout.

TWIST AND SHOUT •• 2 POINTS

Maybe you don't need to shout, but I do want you to twist, a lot and in all different directions. While some machines, like the free motion cable or the cable crossover, require you to use your core muscles to perform the exercise correctly, the best way to implement this tip is to work with your body weight and free weights and avoid machines that artificially isolate muscle groups and function on one plane—front to back, side to side, up and down. A seated hamstring curl is a perfect example. Our bodies don't work like that in the real world; when we train them that way, it's unnatural and inefficient. The more you can exercise "three dimensionally," the more calories you'll burn, and the more fit and functional you'll be.

Here are a few exercises to try:

- Lunges with a Chop (a chop is a straight-arm diagonal motion that you do as you lunge)
- Speed Skaters (leap side to side)
- 180 Jump Squats (squat, then jump and turn airborne 180 degrees, squat in the other direction, and repeat)

- Lateral Burpees (thrust legs out sideways in plank rather than behind you)
- Surfer Get-ups (jump up from a facedown, lying position as if on a surfboard)

If you don't feel well versed enough to trust yourself with multi-dimensional body weight training at first, try working the following classes into your regimen, once a week minimum, to bring yourself up to speed: kickboxing, dance, yoga, or my BODYSHRED.

GET DOWN! • • • 3 POINTS

Good range of motion, or the distance your body moves from one point to another during an exercise, is key both to being function-ally fit and to getting the most out of your workouts. By moving through the full range of motion for each joint, you gain flexibility, mobility, strength, and a better calorie burn.

Here are a few ways you might be cheating your range of motion during your training:

- A squat where you fail to bring your thighs parallel to the ground.
- A biceps curl or lat pull-down where you never fully release the weight back to the start position or straighten the arms.
- A lunge where the rear knee comes only about 6 inches from the floor instead of 2 inches.
- A military dumbbell press where you never fully straighten your arms overhead.

> **SLIM MYTH:**
> **Muscle turns into fat and or fat gets converted to muscle.**
> **FAST FACT:** Just as fat can't trans-form into muscle, muscle won't transform into fat. Building muscle and losing body fat are two com-pletely different processes. You burn body fat and build muscle, but the idea of converting one to the other is about as possible as turning lead into gold.

Of course, if you're extremely tight and can't get all the way down or all the way up, don't injure yourself trying. But if you're mindlessly moving through your workout, phoning it in or just not pushing hard enough, stop cheating yourself. Moving your body those few extra inches will increase your burn during and after your training, while simultaneously creating a far more fit body.

GET UP! •• 2 POINTS

Hop, bound, jump, spring, soar, skyrocket—that's right. I want you to fly, with an advanced fitness technique called plyometrics, or jump training. Although it was first introduced to athletes in the 1960s and 1970s, in the last decade or so, jump training has become a go-to method for improving athletic performance.

Plyo is a form of high-intensity training that can significantly increase your strength, speed, and endurance, allowing you to burn more calories and lose body fat. Additionally, because plyometric training is so strenuous, it increases your metabolic rate or after-burn for hours afterward.

Here's how it works: you perform a high-velocity movement (like a squat jump) that relies on power generated through the "stretch-shortening cycle." A muscle that is stretched before an explosive contraction (recoil) will contract more forcefully and more rapidly. Using a squat-jump as our example, "squatting down" just prior to the jump lowers your center of gravity and slightly stretches the muscles involved. This is a prep phase. Then as you straighten your legs to jump and leave the floor, you ignite more explosion potential due to the recoil you just created with the lowered squat.

Here are some other examples of how to use it in your workout:

- A lunge in which you jump as you straighten your legs.
- Box jumps, where you literally bend your knees and then jump onto a box or platform.

- Push-ups where you thrust your upper body vertically from the lowered (stretched position) with such force that your hands leave the ground.

To clarify and simplify yet again, adding a jump or a hop to your basic fitness exercises will increase the intensity and calorie burn that comes with the added impact. To get the full benefits of plyo and dramatically enhance the effectiveness of the move, be sure to recoil on the landing. You'll get the added benefit of the "stretch-shortening cycle" when you explode out of it. Make sure, too, that you protect yourself from injury by landing softly toe to heel.

One warning: while the physical benefits of plyo with regard to performance and physique are unsurpassed, this type of training is extremely intense. Don't attempt to experiment or exploit this technique unless you already have a moderate to good level of fitness. If you have an injury or health condition, be sure to consult your doctor before engaging in this activity.

BECOME UNSTABLE •• 2 POINTS

Ever look around the gym at all the weird gadgets and apparatuses like disc pillows, BOSU balls, wobble boards, and so on and wonder how to use them? Well, lucky for you, I'm here to tell you: they're there for balance training. In prepping to write this book, however, I did an enormous review of the recent research, comparing balance training on the floor to using any of these gadgets, particularly in conjunction with strength training. I found a host of inconsistencies, indeed rebel-rousing controversies. Basically I found support for my philosophy, which is that you'll be able to train harder and get better results when you stick to solid surfaces and it's your body that becomes imbalanced, not what you're standing on.

I'm not saying that a balance tool won't improve your balance. But if you want to improve muscle strength, muscle stimulation, and muscle engagement—which is what calorie utilization is all about—I want *you* to get unstable, not the platform you're standing on. Exercises that require stabilization utilize more muscles and are far harder than ones that don't; this will help you burn calories, which is what we're after. In addition, balance is an integral part of overall fitness training to improve coordination, athletic skill, and posture. These gizmos and tools are all fine and fun to play with. I'm not saying don't ever use them. Just remember, I'm about efficiency and getting the best use from your time.

Here are some examples of how to get unbalanced in ways that maximize your burn:

Raise a limb. Instead of balancing on both feet and or both arms during an exercise, raise an arm or leg up or off the floor to create instability such as:

- Do push-ups and try raising a leg off the ground as you perform the exercise.
- Do single-leg squats.
- Perform a side lunge, and as you return to the start position, instead of tapping your lunging leg back to the ground, raise it in a knee lift.
- Perform a plank with one arm elevated and out to the side, or extend both an arm and a leg.
- Do single-leg dead lifts with dumbbells (anytime you bend over then stand up again; it also challenges your sensory system).
- Do cable rows standing on one leg instead of two.

The possibilities are endless. Simply assess the exercise you're performing, and see if you can remove one pillar of support.

Platform savvy. This method incorporates using a solid surface, off of which you lift or lower your own body weight (a calorie burner and a core strengthener) while still testing your balance. Here are a few examples:

- Do single-leg step-ups with a knee lift on a bench or high step.
- Stand on a step and rear-lunge off it.
- Place your rear foot on a flat bench, and do stationary lunges.
- Place one foot or both atop a step platform, and do a push-up.

To get the most out of balance training, incorporate the two simple principles above with a body weight or free weight exercise, and you'll take your results to the next level.

AMP UP YOUR CARDIO

INCH UP YOUR INCLINE • • 2 POINTS

All it takes to torch 15 percent more calories on the treadmill is a little incline. Even upping the treadmill to a 5 percent incline and walking can make a huge difference. The higher you go, the more calories you burn at any speed, without tacking more time onto your workout. Here's an example: If a 145-pound woman walks for 30 minutes at 4.0 mph (a solid fitness-walk pace) without an incline, she'll burn 132 calories. If she adds a 5 percent incline, she'll burn 220 calories. Up the incline to 10 percent, she's still walking, but she'll burn 312 calories. Bonus: upping the incline burns approximately the same amount of calories as jogging for 30 minutes on a flat treadmill. So if you aren't able to jog or run, walking on an incline gives you added intensity, added calorie burn, and great muscle conditioning without added impact.

HANDS OFF •• 2 POINTS

Surely you've heard me hollering at contestants on *Biggest Loser* to get their hands off the treadmill, elliptical trainer, or stepper. I do this because *you burn up to 25 percent fewer calories when you hold on.* That's a heck of a lot, right? Now you see why I yell at them! Honestly, if you are gonna spend that time putting in the work, don't you want to maximize your results? So the next time you have a cardio day at the gym, let go of the handrails! Not only does this up your calorie burn and workout challenge, it's a great and intense workout for your core.

DO ARM-POWERED CARDIO •• 2 POINTS

When you're walking, jogging, or running, drive your elbows straight back instead of loosely swinging your arms or letting them hang at your sides. This will instantaneously increase your pace with less leg effort and increase whole-body training and workout efficacy.

SLIM MYTH:

If cardio is part of your training, you won't gain any muscle.

FAST FACT: While performing cardio may make gaining muscle a little harder, it's still possible to get ripped doing it. If "shredding" is your goal and you love your cardio too, just make sure to continue doing resistance training during the week, get adequate nutrients necessary for muscle maintenance, and switch your cardio sessions from longer endurance sessions to shorter sprints. Ever seen the legs of a sprinter? Enough said.

SWITCH IT UP •• 2 POINTS

If you've been toiling on the treadmill and never think about getting on another piece of cardio equipment at the gym, this tip is for you. Every machine will challenge your body differently, and whether you think so or not, it's easy to get accustomed to the same old, same old. To get cross-training benefits, as well as to beat a cardio plateau and bust boredom, use a different machine for each cardio workout. Or get creative and use two or three different machines in the same workout. The time will go by more quickly, and you'll get an amazing workout!

OPTIMIZE OUTDOOR SPACES

TAKE IT TO THE HOOD • 1 POINT

A great way to fend off boredom is to take your workout outdoors. You have everything you need just outside your front door, right in your own neighborhood. You can get a mega burn using your surrounding environment to create your own personal gym. Find a park or wide-open space, and perform old-school calisthenics like jumping jacks, mountain climbers, jump rope, butt kicks, or high knees. Do body weight training like squats, pliés, lunges, push-ups, or sit-ups. You can utilize outdoor props such as a bench, a kid's jungle gym, a wall, a tree, or a lamppost.

Here are some fun ideas:

- Do wall sits on a flat wall.
- Do triceps dips, push-ups, step-ups, or sit-squats on a bench.
- Do lat pull-up rows holding on to a sturdy tree or street pole.
- Do reverse lunges or step-plyos off a curb (not on a busy street!).
- Do pull-ups on playground jungle gym bars.
- For cardio, do HIIT intervals outside, using your blocks as interval definers: walk a block, run a block. Squeeze in any of the above exercises along the way.
- At a park or at the beach, create two markers approximately 50 yards

SLIM MYTH:

Toning shoes actually shape your legs and lift your butt.

FAST FACT: Of course they don't! This notion falls under the category of "if it sounds too good to be true, it is"! Two recent studies from the American Council on Exercise concluded there's "simply no evidence to support the claims that these shoes will help wearers exercise more intensely, burn more calories, or improve muscle strength and tone." The council's Todd Galati found no difference between these special shoes and regular sneakers (other than their prices), noting, "These shoes are not a magic pill." It's the walking that will make a difference in your life—not the shoes.

apart. (One long stride is roughly equal to one yard.) Then sprint from one marker to the other 20 times. Each time you reach a marker, rotate in one of the following exercises: 20 lunges, 20 squats, 20 push-ups, 20 sit-ups, or a plank-hold for 20 seconds. Rest for 30 seconds between intervals.

FEEL THE EARTH MOVE • 1 POINT

Doing your cardio outside can dramatically enhance your burn. Studies show that, thanks to the variations in incline and instability provided by terrain changes (as well as the added resistance from wind or water currents against your body), your heart rate beats an average of 5 to 10 times more per minute when you work out outside. For your next workout, if the weather cooperates, pound the pavement instead of the treadmill. Try road biking instead of going to spin class; run up the bleachers at the local high school stadium instead of using the stepper at your gym. Swim in the ocean instead of in the pool; instead of using the rowing machine, go kayaking on a local river.

ADD IT UP, DROP IT OFF

GIVE YOURSELF 3 POINTS

- Consistency is key.
- Remodel your muscles.
- Stay in motion.
- Put it together.
- Push it good.
- Get down!

GIVE YOURSELF 2 POINTS

- Split it up and take a load off.
- Second time's a charm.
- Angle it!
- Pump it up.
- Mix it up.
- Speed it up.
- Double down.
- Give yourself leverage.
- Twist and shout.
- Get up!
- Become unstable.
- Inch up your incline.
- Hands off.
- Do arm-powered cardio.
- Switch it up.

GIVE YOURSELF 1 POINT

- Dress for the part.
- Do a five-minute warm-up.
- Take it to the hood.
- Feel the earth move.

_____ Total *points* for Chapter 2

_____ Total number of *tips* I'm
incorporating

CHAPTER 3

AT HOME

As I've said, the purpose of this book is to make sure
you're bomb-proof. I want you to have a ridiculous number of strategies in place so you can handle anything and
everything that might otherwise compromise your ability to lose weight and get healthy. With that in mind, it's
imperative we tackle anything that happens in your home
that can affect your weight and wellness. Your home is literally your home base. For this reason we have to be sure
it's rock solid. I'm talking about the groceries you bring
into it, the home gym you might consider constructing for
it, the beauty products you keep in your bathroom, and
even the home cleansers you use. That's right, I'm leaving
no stone unturned. I love you that much! If you're panick-
ing and thinking I'm going to cost you a fortune in this
chapter, think again. You'll probably save money when all
is said and done.

Grocery Shopping

First let's tackle the most obvious hurdle, and that's what's in your kitchen. We talked a lot about diet principles and strategies in Chapter 1, and now it's time to start implementing them.

The food you keep and cook is an integral part of your success, and this section is going to illustrate all the ways to slim down your grocery choices so they subsequently slim you down.

SHOPPING SLIM

THE CENTER WILL INCREASE YOUR CENTER • • • 3 POINTS

This one is as obvious as it gets. Avoid the center aisles as much as you can, and shop the store perimeter, where fresh foods like fruits, vegetables, dairy, meat, and fish are usually located. The center aisles are where the junk food—cookies, chips, breads, cereals, and other tempting nonnecessities—are found.

KEEP YOUR HEAD DOWN • • • 3 POINTS

If you do have to venture into the center aisles for something, look on the bottom shelves. The higher-profit items—the ones that are more highly processed and that are made cheaply with fake, crap ingredients—are placed at eye level. The healthier foods that cost food companies more to produce are usually placed on lower shelves to incentivize you to buy the higher-profit item.

CART IT AROUND • 1 POINT

According to a recent study, published in the *Journal of Marketing Research*, on embodied cognition (the notion that physical movement affects our cognitive function and our decision-making processes), if you walk the aisles of a supermarket with a shopping cart instead of a basket, you're likely to make healthier choices. Basket shoppers are more likely to choose sweets and other empty-calorie foods over healthy and nutritious items, because holding a basket can trigger a desire for instant gratification. But when you're pushing a cart, you're often keeping your arms extended, a body language "repeatedly associated with rejecting undesired objects." So the next time you're at your local market, grab the cart over the basket. And if all else fails, you can burn some calories riding it like a scooter. That's what I always do.

DON'T SHOP WHILE YOU'RE HUNGRY—EVER! • • • 3 POINTS

Do not, under any avoidable circumstances, go grocery shopping when you're hungry. This is a recipe for disaster. Being hungry impairs our judgment and compromises our willpower, leading us to buy too much food and the wrong kinds. Not only is that bad for your diet, it's also bad for your pocketbook. Be sure you put some food in your belly *before* you hit the supermarket.

BE LIKE SANTA • • 2 POINTS

Cheesy title aside, my point is that you should make a grocery list and check it

....

SLIM MYTH:
Fasting is a great way to lose weight.

FAST FACT: Fasting is a sure-fire way to destroy your metabolism. Even though you'll see a temporary weight loss, the key word here is *temporary*. You'll lose weight while fasting, but then when you eat normally again, you'll gain it all back and then some. Here's why: from a biochemical perspective, fasting throws your body into starvation mode. Your body responds by releasing hormones to slow metabolism, cannibalize muscle, and store fat. Fat is needed for survival, while muscle is not. In addition, muscle burns more calories than fat, and when the body is in conservation-of-calories mode, it wants to shed all muscle possible in order to survive. Don't fast, unless it's for a religious purpose that you feel strongly about, and even then you should do it for only a very short period of time.
....

twice. This will allow you to make better decisions, because as you plan out your weekly meals, the unhealthy foods won't be right in front of you, tempting you. In addition, the list becomes a directive, so you aren't wandering aimlessly down those dangerous center aisles undecided, subjecting yourself to fattening impulse-buys.

GO SOLO: DON'T TAKE THE KIDS • • 2 POINTS

If you have little ones in your life, don't take them with you to the market, if you can avoid it. I learned this one the hard way, strolling down the cereal aisle with my two-year-old. She, of course, wanted every box of crap with a cartoon on it, and when I wouldn't put it in the cart, a tantrum ensued. Kids are kids; we are the adults. It's our job to protect them and make healthy decisions for the whole family. Willpower is tough enough to exert for ourselves without the added stress of coping with a tantrum that's wearing you down. Even if your kids are past the "terrible twos" stage, do you really need the pressure of arguments over Froot Loops?

WEAR YOUR SKINNY JEANS • 1 POINT

Ditch your sweats and slide into jeans on your next shopping trip. This will serve as a reminder that you still want to fit in them, and so will incentivize you from succumbing to cravings or buying what you don't need.

SLIMMING FOODS

GO LOW • • 2 POINTS

I mentioned in Chapter 1 that you should be wary of fat-free foods because they have a ton of fillers and junk in them to compensate for their lack of texture and flavor. Conversely, you don't need *all* the fat in the full-fat versions either. We need a certain amount of healthy fat in our diet, but fat is still high in calories (9 calories per gram, as opposed to 4 calories per gram for protein and carbs). For this reason, the low-fat option is optimal; you get the nutritional benefit without the added calories. Choose low-fat milk, low-fat Greek yogurt, low-fat cottage cheese, and leaner cuts of meat.

> **EZ CALORIE CUT**
> For 2 tablespoons of regular mayonnaise, substitute 2 tablespoons of reduced-fat light mayonnaise. **CUT: 83 CALORIES**

BE WHOLESOME • • • 3 POINTS

Get 100 percent whole-grain versions of any and all grains. Your breads, pastas, cereals, baked goods, and of course grain side dishes must be whole. Don't be tricked by the labels *multigrain, seven-grain, twelve-grain,* or *organic flour*. This is important because *100 percent whole-grain* means that neither the nutrients nor the fiber have been removed during processing. Eating whole grains is associated with numerous health benefits, from lowering blood pressure to preventing type 2 diabetes and heart disease. Plus, the fiber content stabilizes our blood sugar and keeps us fuller longer, helping us to eat less. Be sure the front of the package says "100% whole grain" or has the orange "whole grains" stamp on it. If you still aren't sure, check the ingredients list.

Here's a list of common whole grains you can find. For information on each

SLIM MYTH:

If you want to slim down, go gluten-free.

FAST FACT: Unless you're truly allergic to gluten and/or have the autoimmune disorder known as celiac disease (which applies to 1 in 133 Americans, according to the Celiac Disease Foundation), going gluten-free makes no difference. In fact, gluten-free foods often have more calories and less fiber than their gluten counterparts. Plus, gluten-free foods are more expensive. Stick with whole grains as your best choice.

one, what it is, and how to eat it, check out this link to the Whole Grain Council: www.wholegrainscouncil.org/whole-grains-101/whole-grains-a-to-z.

- Amaranth
- Barley
- Buckwheat
- Corn, including whole cornmeal and popcorn
- Millet
- Oats and oatmeal
- Quinoa
- Rice, both brown and colored (such as red, purple, and black)
- Rye
- Teff
- Triticale
- Wheat, including varieties such as spelt, Kamut, durum, bulgur, cracked, and wheat berries
- Wild rice

When you read the package label, all the grains and flours it lists should be preceded by the word *whole*. Suppose you see a package that says "whole wheat." That's considered whole grain, according to the Whole Grain Commission; but unless it says "100% whole grain," chances are the product contains 100 percent refined whole-wheat flour. Obviously, 100 percent whole-grain selections are the best option. Your next best choice is 100 percent whole-wheat flour. Here are some of my favorite 100 percent whole-grain and whole-wheat selections for pastas, breads, and cereals:

Choose from these pastas:

Eden Organic 100% Whole-Wheat Pasta
Eden Organic 100% Whole-Grain Kamut & Quinoa Twisted Pair

Eden Organic 100% Whole-Grain Rye Spirals

Heartland 100% Whole-Wheat Pasta

Hodgson Mill Gluten-free Brown Rice Pasta

Hodgson Mill 100% Whole-Wheat Pasta

Choose from these cereals:

Kellogg's Mini-Wheats

Nature's Path Crunchy Vanilla

Nature's Path Flax Plus Pumpkin Raisin Crunch

Nature's Path Hemp Plus Oatmeal

Nature's Path Heritage Flakes *or* Flax Plus Flakes

Choose from these breads:

EarthGrains 100% Natural 7-Grain

EarthGrains 100% Natural Wheat Berry with Honey

EarthGrains 100% Natural Whole Wheat 100% Stone Ground

Ezekiel brand bread (any)

Nature's Own Organic 24 Grams Whole Grain 100% Whole
    Wheat

Nature's Own 100% Whole Grain

Pepperidge Farm 100% Natural, 15 Grain

Pepperidge Farm 100% Natural, Whole Grain German Dark
    Wheat

Pepperidge Farm 100% Whole Grain, Whole Wheat

Pepperidge Farm Whole Grain Oatmeal

Sara Lee Hearty and Delicious 100% Whole Wheat with
    Honey

Sara Lee Hearty and Delicious 100% Whole Grain

Sara Lee Soft & Smooth 100% Whole Wheat

Sara Lee Soft & Smooth Whole Grain White

Choose from these side dishes:

Amaranth

Barley

Bulgur

Brown rice

Long-grain rice

Quinoa

Wild rice

Choose from these brands:

Arrowhead Mills

Bob's Red Mill

Ezekiel

Grain Place Foods

Nature's Path

You're not limited to the items in the lists above; I just want to give you a little direction. As long as you follow the general guidelines I've outlined, you'll be fine.

GO FISH • 1 POINT

Choosing seafood can be confusing, especially with regard to how it affects your health and your waistline. Here are a few simple rules to follow that will keep you swimming in the right direction without having to fight upstream:

> **EZ CALORIE CUT**
> Love sushi? Instead of a rainbow roll, eat a California roll. **CUT: 128 CALORIES**

- Always go with "wild caught." Many farmed fish are genetically modified, have antibiotics fed to them, and are doused with pesticides. All this crap wreaks havoc on your metabolism, as I established in Chapter 1.

- For the sake of your health, avoid large predatory fish like swordfish and shark; they accumulate more mercury and toxins than other ocean species.

Here's my simple go-to list. All these choices are good, but the starred fishes are the best slim catch, as they're the leanest and lowest in calories:

Abalone	Pacific pollock
Alaskan wild salmon (fresh, frozen, or canned)	Pacific rockfish
Anchovies	Rainbow trout
Atlantic char*	Sablefish
Atlantic herring	Sardines*
Black sea bass	Snapper*
Clams (steamers)	Sole*
Grouper*	Stone, Kona, and Dungeness crab
Haddock*	Tilefish*
Halibut*	Tuna* (white albacore, line caught from the United States or Canada, canned, in water)
Mahi mahi*	
Oysters/mussels	
Pacific cod*	
Pacific halibut*	

DON'T CUT CORNERS • 1 POINT

When buying fruits and veggies, make sure they aren't precut. Produce that has been precut has been exposed to the air and is subsequently being "oxidized." The fruit or vegetable is losing its nutrients and aging. Have you ever seen an apple an hour after you've taken a bite from it? It's all brown, right? That's oxidization at work for you.

Don't be lazy. I mean really, how hard is it to eat it whole or cut it yourself? Precut fruit is more expensive and has fewer metabolism-boosting nutrients.

JUDGE FOOD BY ITS COVER • 1 POINT

When you have to hack through layers of packaging and plastic to get to your food, it's most likely bad for you. Plus, much of that plastic packaging is loaded with endocrine-disrupting perfluorochemicals (PFCs). Companies aren't required to phase out the use of these harmful PFCs until 2015, but you can do it now. Try the strategy in the next tip as the ultimate alternative.

EXHAUST THE CASHIER • 1 POINT

Buy foods without bar codes. Think about it. Anything healthy, fresh, and minimally processed has no extra packaging or bar code. Veggies and fruits; grains, beans, and seeds from bulk bins; and meat—they come naturally, without a bar code. So make it your mission to wear out the cashier by having him or her look up the cost of all your healthy food choices!

KICK THE CAN • 1 POINT

The inside of many food cans is laced with a toxic coating called bisphenol A (BPA). Numerous studies have shown the effects of this dangerous chemical on our health. Research also suggests that BPA is directly linked to childhood obesity. Don't think you're off the hook, grown-up! It makes adults fat, too. And here's how: BPA can act like the female hormone estrogen, and when it's out of whack, it can throw off our endocrine system and trigger our fat cells to grow. Look for foods packed in glass jars instead of cans; get veggies fresh or frozen; buy beans from bulk bins. If you must buy canned, try to make sure the label says "BPA-free" before you purchase the product.

MAKE A CLEAN CUT •• 2 POINTS

As we established in Chapter 1, the quality of the food you eat is critical to cracking *Slim for Life*. However, when it comes to meat, it's not just the quality that matters—the cut of the meat matters too. Even though something may be healthy, it doesn't mean that it's low in calories. Here are the slimmest cuts of meat for all you carnivores out there seeking to look svelte:

- **Pork**—loin chops, sirloin chops, and center loin chops
- **Poultry**—breasts
- **Beef**—loin and round cuts, like choice or select sirloin (not prime sirloin). Specific cuts made from sirloin include tri-tip roast, tri-tip steak, and top sirloin steak. (Top sirloin is very lean at 5 grams of fat per 4-ounce serving.)
- **Lamb**—shank or leg of lamb, lamb chop, and lamb roast

DON'T BE TRICKED BY FOOD MARKETERS

Most of the advice in this book is pretty straightforward, but here's where it can get confusing: not all processed foods are bad for you. The term *processed* has a broad definition. It essentially means "prepared for ease of consumption." Frozen vegetables or 100 percent whole-grain oatmeal are processed foods, and I'd never tell you not to eat them. The way to differentiate the healthy and slimming from the disease-inducing and fattening is to learn what to look for on the labels. That's what I'm going to show you now: how to decode labels and dodge food-marketing trickery so you never get fooled or confused again.

FOOD LABELS 101

SERVE IT UP • • • 3 POINTS

Many food labels hide the true amount of calories in that food by splitting up servings. For example, if you buy a regular-size bottle of Snapple (which I hope to God you never do), it's highly unlikely that you planned on sharing it. Common sense dictates that the whole bottle is one serving. The label says it's 120 calories per serving, which sounds fine. Look more closely at that label, however, and you'll see that this one bottle is meant to serve 2.5 people. Drink that bottle, and you'll be swigging down 300 calories. You just drank almost your entire calorie allotment for a meal, without even eating a sandwich. Moral of the story: when you read a food label, always check the number of servings first, *then* the number of calories per serving. The serving size is the amount you would have to eat to ingest the nutrition shown on the rest of the food label, no more, no less.

KEEP IT SHORT AND SIMPLE • • • 3 POINTS

Buy food with as few ingredients listed on the label as possible. If you're wondering how many ingredients are too much, keeping them to five and under is a good rule of thumb.

CHECK: ONE, TWO, THREE • • • 3 POINTS

Ingredients are listed in order of their quantity in the food. So the top three ingredients are pretty much all you're eating. And while you might think something is healthy because it has pomegranate in it (or some other fruit or vegetable), the top three ingredients might also include high-fructose corn syrup, enriched flour, and cornstarch. Don't be deceived. If the top three ingredients are crap, then the food is crap. Put it back and make a healthier choice.

BE A MATCHMAKER • • • 3 POINTS

Have you ever played with a little kid who matches up the same animals or the same shapes in a puzzle? This is essentially what I want you to do when you look at ingredients on a label—match up the ones that are the same thing, even if they have a different name. One of the most common label deception tricks is to list sugars as different ingredients so that sugar doesn't appear in the top three. For example, the label for a high-sugar food might list sucrose, high-fructose corn syrup, corn syrup solids, brown sugar, dextrose, and other sugar ingredients to keep sugar out of the top position on the ingredients list. So if you see a label that lists two separate forms of sugar, put it back on the shelf on principle alone, not just because it will make you fat.

SAY IT LOUD • • • 3 POINTS

If you can't pronounce it, don't buy it. Chances are that if an ingredient is not a common food or spice, then it's a GMO or a manufactured, fake, chemical ingredient. It's also likely an obesogen. You don't want it. Your body doesn't need it. Let it go, and pass it by.

GET OUT YOUR DECODER RING • • • 3 POINTS

It's amazing how clever these marketing people can be, and they work in ways you would never imagine are even legal.

Here's how to read between the lines and sniff out the BS.

- **"Gluten free."** Just because something is gluten free doesn't mean it's low calorie or good for you. Gluten is a protein found in wheat or foods processed with wheat. Unless you

have celiac disease or you've been tested for gluten sensitivity, you don't need to worry about it. In fact, as I said on page
74, gluten-free foods are often higher in calories, have less
fiber, and are more expensive. Don't buy into the hype.

- **"All natural."** This food claim literally means nothing. Sure, it
brings to mind thoughts of fresh, minimally processed food.
Many people even confuse this claim with "organic," but
they're not even remotely the same. The word *natural* has no
regulatory meaning, while *organic* does. Food manufacturers
can put "all natural" on a label even when the ingredients are
not at all natural. Be sure to read exactly what is in the product before you buy it.

- **"Fortified."** Lots of processed foods are "fortified" with fiber,
omega-3s, calcium, and the like to make you think they're
healthy. The problem is that the quality of the nutrients used
is often garbage. Take inulin, for example, a cheap fiber processed from chicory root. A manufacturer may claim that
since its product is "fortified" with inulin, it will help you get
your daily fiber requirements. Studies have shown, however,
that inulin doesn't lower cholesterol or create feelings of fullness the way 100 percent whole-grain fiber does. Similarly,
the omega-3 that is used to "fortify" food is often ALA, which
pales in comparison to the varieties that come from fish like
DHA and EPA. Again, fortified foods are usually junk that's
been enriched with cheap versions of vitamins and minerals
to mislead you into thinking they're healthy. Don't fall for it.

- **"Fruit Flavor."** There's no fruit in fruit flavoring. Although the
label might say that a food contains "natural flavors," this just
means that at some point it originated from a plant or animal.
Nowadays food scientists create flavors using bacteria and
call them, say, "natural strawberry flavor" (sans strawberries).
Why do food manufacturers use them, you ask? Because
they're cheaper.

- **"Heart Healthy."** This claim is often used on products that contain corn oil. If you look closely at the packaging, though, you'll see the fine print, which says it all: "The FDA concludes there is little scientific evidence supporting this claim." Corn oil is actually high in omega-6, a fat that studies in the *British Journal of Nutrition,* among others, have linked to obesity and high cholesterol.

IF IT SOUNDS TOO GOOD TO BE TRUE, IT'S BS • • • 3 POINTS

Here's an amazing con that food manufacturers run that can lead you down the road to ruin: they round down. Legally they're able to say that a food contains "0 grams of trans fats" or "0 calories" when the food is actually loaded with trans fats or calories. This is my all-time favorite example: back when I was still an idiot eating a ton of "fat-free" diet foods, I fell in love with I Can't Believe It's Not Butter spray. I put it on *everything.* I sprayed it on popcorn, cooked eggs in it, and smothered my toast with it. You name it—I found a way to flavor some crappy diet food with it. I mean, why wouldn't I? It tasted just like butter, and it had zero calories and zero grams of trans fats—right? *Wrong!*

I looked at the label. The top ingredient listed was hydrogenated soybean oil. Now, I'm not a genius, but it doesn't take a genius to know that oil is not calorie free. Having been around the block a tiny bit at that point, I knew that *hydrogenated* was also synonymous with *trans fat.* How could this be? Confused and pissed, I called the food manufacturer, and the truth came out. Because there were 0.9 calories in one spray and a serving size was one spray, they were legally able to round down. So they were saying that it was zero calories and zero grams of trans fats, even though there were about 1,200 calories in that tiny bottle—nearly all of which were from trans fats.

To sum up my long story, if a food claim sounds too good to be true, investigate and get to the truth. If you don't have time but you're in doubt, ditch it. Make a different, more clearly healthy choice.

BE SALT SAVVY • • • 3 POINTS

Although sodium is a transient mineral with zero calories, it *can* adversely affect your weight. Some studies suggest that sodium can even influence cortisol levels in the body (and high levels of cortisol have been linked to increased belly fat). Also, foods that are high in sodium are usually highly processed and high in calories. Excess sodium is bad for your blood pressure and makes you bloated. So with this mineral, a little goes a long, long way. Make sure that your food choices have fewer milligrams of sodium per serving than calories per serving. And as a general rule of thumb, people 50 years of age and under should aim to consume no more than 2,000 milligrams of sodium per day. Those 51 and older should shoot for no more than 1,500 daily milligrams.

BE SUGAR SAVVY • • • 3 POINTS

Large amounts of sugar are bad for your diet, but not solely because processed foods that are high in sugar are also usually high in calories. Sugar-laden foods also cause insulin levels to spike. These spikes will crash your blood sugar, lead to hunger, and so promote fat storage. To avoid this problem, for any packaged food, keep your sugar intake below 5 grams per serving.

BE LIKE GRANDMA—GET YOUR FIBER • • • 3 POINTS

Did your grandmother ever tell you how important it is to get enough fiber in your diet? Mine was obsessed with making sure we kids ate our fiber each day. Grandmothers are smart. You know that I want you to buy grain products that are 100 percent whole grain. But if, for some reason, that isn't an option, make sure that the product you choose has at least 2 grams of fiber per 100 calories. Remember, fiber is important because it helps stabilize your blood sugar and fill you up, diminishing your hunger and inhibiting a tendency to overeat.

....

Get Cooking

All right, now that you've brought the healthy food home from the grocery store, just what the heck do you do with it? It's not enough that the food is intrinsically good for you. Any healthy food can be made unhealthy in the way it's prepared.

Let's make sure that your cooking strategies stack the scales in your favor (or in this case, unstack them).

SLIM CHEFFING

BREAK THE RULES • • • 3 POINTS
Many recipes don't have weight loss and health as their main focus. So don't always follow a recipe—modify it to meet your needs. That doesn't mean you have to sacrifice flavor. In most cases, though, a large amount of the salt, sugar, and fat that a recipe calls for is unnecessary. You can cut out the extra, and it will still taste good, I promise. Try these approaches to make your dishes way healthier while still retaining their flavor:

- Cut out a third of the fat.
- Cut the sugar in half.
- Cut the salt in half. Then continue to reduce it slightly each time you prepare a favorite recipe, until you have gone as low as possible while still retaining the food's flavor.

SWAP IT OUT • • • 3 POINTS

Instead of reducing the amount of unhealthy ingredients, you're going to *replace* them with healthier, lower-calorie ones:

- For savory dishes, instead of using butter or oil, try low-fat, low-sodium chicken broth.
- For baked goods, instead of using butter, replace it with:
    - ✓ unsweetened applesauce
    - ✓ mashed bananas
    - ✓ prunes
    - ✓ olive oil or coconut oil (They're not lower in calories, but they provide health benefits that corn oil doesn't.)
- For baked goods, instead of using frosting, use a meringue or low-fat yogurt.
- Instead of using cream, try coconut milk (from the carton not the can).
- Instead of using jam or syrup, use puréed fruit.
- Instead of using full-fat sour cream or mayonnaise, use low-fat yogurt.
- Ditch the sugar and instead use:
    - ✓ unsweetened apple sauce
    - ✓ agave
    - ✓ organic maple syrup (It's not lower in calories, but at least it has health benefits.)
    - ✓ raw honey (Again, it's not lower in calories, but it offers health benefits.)
    - ✓ stevia

SLIM MYTH:

You should only eat egg whites, not the yolks.

FAST FACT: For years now (I mean like years and years), egg yolks have been demonized, supposedly being terrible for your cholesterol. We now know that that's not the case. Eggs won't affect your cholesterol balance unless they're fried in butter and served with bacon. In fact, one study at the University of Connecticut found that the fat in egg yolks helped reduce LDL ("bad") cholesterol. And if that's not enough to persuade you, the yolk contains most of the vitamins and minerals in the egg, plus half its protein.

✓ xylitol (It's as sweet as table sugar with 40 percent fewer calories and 75 percent fewer carbohydrates; it's not thought to spike blood sugar.)

✓ erythritol (This sugar alcohol contains almost zero calories and has no effect on blood sugar; it's primarily used in baking.)

- Replace white flour with:
  ✓ spelt flour
  ✓ whole-wheat flour
  ✓ almond flour

SPICE IT UP •• 2 POINTS

Using dry rubs to season your meats is a great way to save calories, as they help you avoid fattening dressings and sauces. You can purchase many good premade rubs. Mrs. Dash is a great brand and it's sodium free. If you feel like putting in a little extra effort, here are some good options you can throw together yourself:

> **EZ CALORIE CUT**
> For 8 ounces of chicken fingers, substitute an 8-ounce grilled chicken breast.
> **CUT: 272 CALORIES**

JERK RUB (RIBS, CHICKEN, OR FISH)

1 tablespoon onion powder

1 tablespoon brown sugar

1 tablespoon dried thyme, crushed

1½ teaspoons allspice

½ teaspoon salt

1 teaspoon fresh cracked black pepper

½ teaspoon ground nutmeg

½ teaspoon ground cinnamon

½ teaspoon ground cloves

¼ teaspoon ground red pepper

SOUTHERN RUB (PORK)

2 tablespoons paprika

1 teaspoon coarse ground black pepper

1 teaspoon white pepper

½ teaspoon onion powder

½ teaspoon garlic salt

1 teaspoon chili powder

1 tablespoon dark brown sugar

1 teaspoon dry mustard

CITRUS SPLASH (CHICKEN OR TURKEY)

¼ cup fresh rosemary leaves

6–8 cloves garlic, roughly chopped

zest of one orange

zest of one lemon

2 tablespoons fresh thyme

2 tablespoons orange juice

1 pinch salt

CHILI (BEEF AND CHICKEN)

2 dried chipotle peppers (use 3 to heat it up a little)

3 tablespoons black pepper

2 tablespoons dried oregano

1 tablespoon dried cilantro leaves

1 bay leaf

1 teaspoon cumin

1 teaspoon onion powder

1 teaspoon ground dry orange peel

CHEW MINT GUM • 1 POINT

How many times have you been cooking and sampled a bite here, licked a spoon there? (As a kid, I loved to lick the beaters when my mom baked something. As an adult, I still look forward to doing that, but my kids won't let me near 'em.) Those calories really add up. A simple way to avoid this excess calorie accumulation is to chew gum—preferably mint. Think about it—if you're chewing mint gum, you're probably not going to be as inclined to have a nibble of goat cheese from the heirloom tomato salad you're preparing. Most gums are loaded with chemicals and crap like artificial sweeteners and colors, but there's one brand that's clean that I approve of completely: it's called Spry. Give it a try when you're getting your chef on.

ADD TO YOUR RECIPE DECK • 1 POINT

I want you to try a new recipe every month. This will help you expand your library of healthy options and keep you from getting bored with your food. Healthy recipes are easy to find. *Cooking Light, Shape,* and *Women's Health* are great sources for healthy, low-calorie, tasty options.

START FLASHING •• 2 POINTS

While I absolutely never want you to fry your food, there's a way to cheat so you don't break your calorie budget. When it comes to fried foods, what affects your weight isn't the amount of oil you *cook* the food in—it's the amount of *time* it sits in that oil. The amount of fat and calories that are absorbed in frying food is a function of time, not quantity. If you absolutely must fry something—say, for a special event—here's how you do it: Use an oil that has a high smoke point, like avocado, safflower, or sunflower oil. Put enough oil in the pan to submerge the food. Heat the oil until it's boiling, around 400 degrees Fahrenheit. Submerge the food for 30 to 60 seconds, remove it, and pat off the excess oil.

One caveat—when it comes to chicken or turkey, you need to precook the meat before you flash-fry it to make sure it's cooked through and spends minimal time in the oil. Here's how: Lay out all the chicken chunks on a microwave-safe plate and season both sides. Place the plate in the microwave and cook on high for 1 minute and 30 seconds. Remove the plate, and turn each piece of chicken over. Microwave again on high until the chunks are just cooked through, about another 1 minute and 30 seconds to 2 minutes depending on your microwave. Let the chicken cool to room temperature. Then coat it with your topping, like egg whites and wheat flour. Finally, flash-fry the chicken or turkey for roughly 30 seconds per side.

DRY OFF •• 2 POINTS
The way you cook your food can have a dramatic impact on your physique. The goal is to use as little oil or butter as possible to save on unneeded calories. As I've already mentioned, avoid frying your food; the healthiest methods are baking, broiling, grilling, and steaming. When it comes to a sauté, technique is everything. A little bit of oil is healthy (try olive, grapeseed, flaxseed, or coconut), but a lot is not. If you can afford it, cook your food in titanium pots and pans. Titanium is nontoxic, unlike Teflon, and it's nonstick, so you won't need much oil or butter to grease it. It's a bit pricey but well worth it if you've got the spare cash.

CHILL OUT AND SAVE CALORIES •• 2 POINTS
You may have seen your mom or grandma do this, or maybe you do it yourself. Chill stews and gravies, then skim the congealed fat off the top. By doing so, you'll save your arteries from excess saturated fats and can shave off up to 100 calories per serving.

KEEP IT FIRM •• 2 POINTS
My gosh, I've written a lot of innuendo into this chapter's tip titles. At least I know I'm keeping your attention. When you make pasta, cook it al dente. You will then digest it more slowly, which helps to control the rate at which it releases insulin into your bloodstream.

This slowed release will subsequently help stabilize blood sugar and inhibit fat storage.

STOCK UP SLIMLY

BUILD A TOOLBOX • • 2 POINTS
Be proactive and prepared by stocking your kitchen with skinny tools. I'm referring to items that will help you count and save calories.

- **Keep a kitchen scale handy.** I know—weighing out your portions sounds so tedious, and it makes eating more a chore than a pleasure. But accuracy is critical for calorie counting, and you're on a slim mission here, after all. Here's the good news: much as with food journaling, you likely won't need to do this for more than several weeks, as you'll eventually learn how to accurately eyeball portion sizes. And this skill, once you learn it, will be a nifty one to have when you're eating out.

  Using a kitchen scale to measure portions will give you a far more accurate frame of reference than using your hand (your fist equals 1 cup, your thumb equals 1 oz., and so on). It's an unreliable method. Think about it—everyone's fist, thumb, or palm is a different size. It will give you a ballpark, but that's it— and most people who use the hand method are eating out-of-the-ballpark portions. Once you see what 5 ounces really looks like, because you've truly measured it, you'll be able to judge far more accurately in the future when you don't have it handy.

- **Get yourself a pack of measuring cups.** Don't just pour cereal out of a box and hope you measured the serving size accurately. Measure out how much you're going to eat, for the same reason you should use a kitchen scale—so you can truly control how much you're eating.

- **Get an oil mister.** In case you weren't able to get those titanium pans I just talked about in "Dry off," an oil mister will allow you to grease your pan with as few calories as possible.

- **Buy a steamer.** Steaming is a great method for slim food preparation. Worried about flavor? Don't be—there are plenty of herbs and spices that you can use to perk up your food and satisfy your taste buds. That leads me to my next suggestion.

- **Scoop up an herb mill.** This little bad boy will help you shred fresh herbs to season your food. You can just use dried herbs, but fresh have more phytonutrients and less salt.

- **Get glass storage containers.** This is so you don't store or reheat your food in plastic. Chemicals in plastic can leach into the food and disrupt your hormone balance and metabolism. While certain plastics are safer than others, why take the chance? Just use glass containers for your food. (A plastic top is okay, as long as it doesn't touch the food.)

- **Get yourself a muffin tin.** No, it's not so you can eat muffins. Muffin tins are great for making small portions of your more fattening foods like quiches, plus they're great for portioning out side dishes. We use them regularly in our home to store healthy fruit and veggie purées for the kids as well as ourselves. You can always freeze any extra for grab-and-go meals or snacks.

KEEP ESSENTIALS ON HAND • • • 3 POINTS

Always make sure to keep healthy essentials handy and stocked in your pantry and refrigerator. This way you can whip up something healthy at a whim, or grab it and go, if need be. Here are some good options to stock up on.

IN THE PANTRY MUST-HAVES

snack-pack-size dry roasted almonds

oatmeal

quinoa (high in protein, cooks quickly)

100 percent whole-grain bread

whole-grain crackers

whole-grain pasta

balsamic vinegar

organic mustard

extra-virgin olive oil or coconut butter

salsa

low-sodium broth

low-sodium line-caught tuna or salmon packed in water
   (canned or in a pouch)

baked tortilla chips

popchips, a 100-calorie snack bag (my personal favorite)

almond butter

canned beans: black, garbanzo, adzuki

brown rice

low-sodium tomatoes (canned)

herbs and spices (such as salt-free lemon pepper, Italian
   seasoning, dry mustard, chili pepper, cinnamon)

HAVE COLD AND READY IN THE FRIDGE

Horizon organic low-fat cheese sticks

small, organic, low-fat Greek yogurts

seasonal fruit

hummus

carrot sticks

turkey slices

head of organic lettuce

berries (frozen, or fresh if in season)

hard-boiled eggs (Boil a dozen eggs and keep them in the
   fridge; they'll last for up to a week after cooking if you keep
   the shells on. Use them to make egg salad, or to add protein
   to a salad or another dish. Or grab one, peel, and go, for a
   great, quick protein pick-me-up.)

....

Get Your Burn On

CALORIE CRUSHERS

I get it, you're busy. Your schedule gets packed with work and family
obligations, and the gym is always the first thing to get cut from
your day. I do this myself. You get overwhelmed, and in the short
term it seems like the most expendable item on that crazy-long
to-do list. After all, you have to make money and take care of your
loved ones, right? Yes, you do, but that doesn't mean it's okay to
stop taking care of you, too. You must make time for yourself and
your health.

One way I manage to do it is by fitting my fitness in at home.
That saves me the drive time to and from the gym, which can be
anywhere from 30 to 60 minutes. Plus, at home there's no check-in,
stuffing clothes in a locker, waiting for a class, or waiting for equipment to become available.

Sometimes we aren't able to leave the house because we're
watching kids or tending to other obligations, but a killer home
workout is within your reach. Try these following action plans,
which are designed to remove all conceivable reasons or excuses for
letting anything keep you from your workout.

SLIP A DISC ... ••• 3 POINTS

... Into your DVD player! Fitness DVDs are a great, affordable way to get your burn on with a fitness professional in the privacy of your own home. Most require minimal equipment, and the exercises can be done in a supersmall space if need be. Invest about fifty bucks (the cost of a personal trainer for a one-hour session) and buy ten used DVDs for your fitness library. The variety will keep you from getting bored and will help you get your daily moves in and on.

BE NEAT AT HOME

What You Need to Know About Non-Exercise Activity Thermogenesis, or NEAT

The calorie burn that comes with everyday activities and nonformal exercise habits was first identified by James Levine, M.D., a prominent researcher at the Mayo Clinic. His research has shown that adding more NEAT to your day can help you burn extra calories. Check out my tip "Fidget" on page 207. Dr. Levine's work suggests that fidgeting is a "NEAT" means to supercharge your slim!

- The next time you mop or vacuum, crank the music and get your heart rate up by dancing.
- Trade your power mower for a push version.
- Instead of using a leaf-blower, sweep the drive or rake the leaves.
- Wash windows by hand.
- Wash your car yourself instead of taking it to the car wash.
- Garden your heart out—pull weeds, trim trees, and plant seasonal flowers and veggies.
- Play fetch with your pooch.
- Balance challenge: When you're prepping food, cooking, folding laundry, or even brushing your teeth, stand on one foot for a minute, then switch to the other foot and repeat.

GRAB A CHAIR • 1 POINT

No, don't sit in it—that's gotten us into enough trouble. Use it as a fitness tool.

It's one of many fitness tools that we have within reach without even realizing it.

Here are a few workout items that are likely to be available in or around your home and neighborhood:

- *Stairs.* Most homes and apartment buildings have stairs. I use them a lot when I can't get out of the house. Simply climb up and down the stairs—even if it's only for 20 minutes. It's nearly as good as the expensive step machine at the gym.
- *Tables or chairs.* You can do step-ups on a stable coffee table or sturdy kitchen chair. You can use them for bench-dips to work your triceps. You can put your heels on top of them, lie back, and do pelvic thrusts. You can even use a chair as a weight if necessary. Try raising it for shoulder presses, chest presses, or biceps curls.
- *Paper plates or hand towels.* These products are great for doing slide work on a wooden or cement floor. They'll create a slippery surface where you can do ab work, leg work, and chest work. There are some great exercise examples on YouTube. Just search for "towel workout" for instructions. Just be careful because of the slipperiness.

IF YOU BUILD IT, YOU'LL USE IT • 1 POINT

Make your own home gym. Although this might seem daunting, time consuming, and expensive, it doesn't have to be any of these things. If you think you don't have the room, you'd be surprised by how little space you actually need. If you aren't able to designate a room to be your home gym, simply create an 8-by-8-foot space to work in (move your coffee table out of the way if you have to) and bring in some simple, very minimal pieces of equipment.

Here's what you'll need:

Your own body. This is your most valuable tool when it comes to exercise, especially when working out at home. There's next to nothing you can't work with body weight alone. To get you started:

- **Buns and thighs.** Do squats, lunges, sumo squats, side lunges, dead lifts, leg lifts, step-ups.
- **Chest, shoulders, and triceps.** Do push-ups, downward-facing dogs, pike push-ups, triceps dips.
- **Back.** Do Supermans, body rows (put a broomstick across two chair seats, lie under it, grab it with an underhand grip, and pull yourself up).
- **Abs.** Do sit-ups, crunches, reverse crunches, bicycle crunches, plank, side plank, leg raises, hollow man (lie face up, arms at sides, palms up, legs extended and together; lift head, shoulders, and legs a few inches off the floor and hold for 30 seconds, "hollowing out" your belly).
- **Cardio.** Do butt kicks, high knees, mountain climbers, jog in place, jumping jacks, skaters.

A pair of adjustable dumbbells. Grab yourself a pair of dumbbells that adjust from 3 to 8 pounds. You can buy some used on eBay for about ten dollars. They allow you to add resistance to many of the exercises listed above, and they open another slew of exercise possibilities to you. You can do rows for your back, flys for your chest, military presses and front and lateral raises for your shoulders, triceps extensions and kickbacks, biceps curls for your arms, and chops (diagonal swings down and across your body) to challenge your core. While it's true that you can use water bottles or candlesticks in place of dumbbells, use them only as a last resort (like when you're traveling and staying in a hotel that has no gym). These things are not meant for fitness so the weight isn't evenly distributed, they're weird to hold, and as a result they can slip from your hand.

A resistance tube. Tubes aren't completely necessary if you have dumbbells, but these elasticized items are so cheap to own, why not add one to your equipment collection? Tubes are interchangeable with bands—it's just that one comes with handles (tubes) and the other is flat and doesn't (bands). They're light and easy to travel with, too. Typically tubes can play the role that cables do at the gym. You can hook a tube under a sofa leg and do seated rows. Wrap it around a post and do cable chest presses or flys. Get an Xergym door attachment (you can purchase it at www.sprifitness.com) and insert it above shoulder height between the hinge side of the door and the door jam to do lat pulldowns. Stand on the tube and do biceps curls, military presses, or triceps extensions—the possibilities are nearly endless.

A yoga mat. I can't recommend that you grab a used one, but having a yoga mat to work out on is important, especially if you have a hard floor. If you really can't afford this addition to your tool kit, lay down two bath towels for padding when you do floor exercises.

A jump rope. This one is pretty self-explanatory. Jumping rope is a cardio calorie-scorcher.

That's pretty much it.

If you have some extra cash, there are two higher-ticket items I'd recommend: a piece of cardio equipment and an exercise bench.

> ### SLIM MYTH:
> ### Lifting weights will make you bulky.
>
> **FAST FACT:** Weight training is great for fat burning and muscle maintenance. Lifting heavy weights, in particular, has a direct effect on raising your resting metabolism, and it boosts calorie burn by approximately 105 calories per day, for up to 3 days after a workout. This afterburn is one huge reason why every woman should regularly strength-train. Women have fewer muscle fibers than men and significantly fewer muscle-building hormones like testosterone. For a woman to get bulky from weights, she would have to be doing Olympic lifts and power-lifting extremely heavy weights while simultaneously eating a massive calorie surplus.

The bench is great for everything from dumbbell chest presses to step-ups to dumbbell rows; it provides you with a stable platform that won't get scuffed up like a coffee table or kitchen chair. For the days you just aren't in the mood to jump around or put yourself through the paces, an incline treadmill is great for getting in a quick burn. You can do it while you watch your favorite shows or get in a quick jog when It's snowing outside. It will give you versatility and convenience. I'd avoid the recumbent bike and elliptical machines, as they don't burn as many calories as the treadmill does.

Clean Products

Removing chemicals and toxins from your food is essential to getting and staying slim. But do you know why it's important to do so with your home products, too? Much of what you put *on* your body gets absorbed *into* your body through your skin. The chemicals and toxins in your cleaning, hygiene, and beauty products can actually make you sick and fat by disrupting your endocrine system. Bummer, right? I'm about to teach you how to fix this problem by greening your routine in affordable ways. You'll get slim, save the planet some, and save money.

THE GREEN HOME

When it comes to home cleaning products like dish soap and detergent, you don't need harsh chemicals to get the job done. In fact, I've asked my favorite green expert Caroline Howell, owner of Green Beanie (www.greenbeanie.net), to recommend her picks for best green cleaning products. Now, these products can get costly, so if money is an issue, keep reading. She'll show you how to make your own at home for pennies.

USE GREEN BRANDS •• 2 POINTS

Bona Hardwood Floor Cleaner

EarthFirst Bath Tissue

EarthFirst Dinner Napkins

EarthFirst Facial Tissue

Ecover Dishwasher Tablets

Ecover Laundry Detergent

Method Furniture Polish

Mrs. Meyer's Liquid Hand Soap

Mrs. Meyer's Powder Surface Scrub

Seventh Generation Natural Dish Liquid

Seventh Generation 100% Paper Towels

Seventh Generation Toilet Bowl Cleaner

Seventh Generation 100% Recycled Bathroom Tissue

Simple Green All Purpose Cleaner

Simple Green Carpet Cleaner

USE HOMEMADE CLEANING ESSENTIALS •• 2 POINTS

- White vinegar is a popular household cleanser, effective for killing most mold, bacteria, and germs, due to its high level of acidity. Cleaning with this vinegar is a smart way to avoid using harsh chemicals. Just mix an equal solution of water and vinegar in a spray bottle, and go to town. It's great for anything you'd use Windex on. You'll also be glad to know that it's environmentally friendly and very economical.

- Baking soda, like vinegar, is nontoxic, multipurpose, and cheap. Simply mix ¼ cup baking soda with 1 quart warm water. It's easiest if you use it in a spray bottle, then wipe the area clean. It does everything from unclogging drains to cleaning pots and pans to removing odors in your fridge. You can also use borax or washing soda, which are slightly stronger than baking soda. Both work well to brighten clothes and lift stains.

- Lemon juice has a pleasant aroma, cuts grease, polishes, and can be used to dissolve soap scum and hard water deposits. Lemon is a great substance to clean and shine brass and copper. Try mixing lemon juice with vinegar or baking soda to make cleaning pastes. Cut a lemon in half and sprinkle baking soda on the cut section of the lemon. Use the lemon to scrub dishes, surfaces, and stains. Be aware that lemon juice can act like a bleach, so test it on a hidden area before putting it everywhere.

- Olive oil is a great natural wax and polish agent for metal or wood. Simply mix 1 cup of olive oil with ½ cup of lemon juice, then start polishing.

- Hydrogen peroxide is an antibacterial and antiviral agent, so it makes sense to use it as a household cleaner. It does take time to work, however, so when you spray it on, leave it for about a minute before wiping it off from whatever you're cleaning. You can use it on everything from toilets to mildewed showers to countertops. Plus, it safely and naturally bleaches and whitens clothing.

- Salt is a natural abrasive that's nontoxic, cheap, and easy to find. Use rock salt or sea salt for tough scrubbing jobs, but don't use it on stainless steel as it may leave scratches.

BE NATURALLY BEAUTIFUL

When it comes to hygiene and beauty, natural and clean is the only way to go. It's ironic that people pay hundreds of dollars on beauty products loaded with chemicals that will age them, disrupt their metabolic function, and possibly induce disease in their bodies. It's all so unnecessary. There are a ton of natural products without harmful chemicals that you can use, as well as home recipes that can replace these toxin-filled products and keep your body functioning optimally. My personal makeup artist and green beauty expert Paige Padgett (www.paigepadgett.com) has put together a list of products and natural ingredients for you to use to beautify. They'll help keep you hot, slim, and healthy. (Notice, I'm giving you big points for these. That's how seriously I take this topic. Taking the chemicals out of your products will make an enormous difference in the long run with regard to your metabolism and your overall health.)

USE THE CLEAN HYGIENE, SKIN CARE, AND BEAUTY BRANDS PAIGE LOVES • • • 3 POINTS

Amala—http://www.amalabeauty.com

Beauty Without Cruelty—http://www.beautywithout cruelty.com

Burt's Bees—http://www.burtsbees.com

California Baby—http://www.californiababy.com

Derma e—http://www.dermae.com/fc_portals/cgibin/ fccgi.exe?w3exec=dfc.portal

Desert Essence—https://www.desertessence.com

Dr. Hauschka—http://www.drhauschka.com

Duchess Marden—http://www.duchessmarden.com

Eccobella—http://www.eccobella.com

Intelligent Nutrients—http://www.intelligentnutrients.com

Jane Iredale—http://www.janeiredale.com

Juice Beauty—http://www.juicebeauty.com

Kjaer Weis—http://kjaerweis.com

Nude Skin Care—http://www.nudeskincare.com

Pangea Organics—http://pangeaorganics-store.sparkart.net

Pratima—http://www.pratimaskincare.com

Primitive Makeup—http://primitivemakeup.com

Revolution Organics—http://www.revolutionorganics.com

Suk-i—http://www.sukipure.com

Tata Harper—http://www.tataharperskincare.com

Terra Firma—http://terrafirmacosmetics.com

Vapour Organics—http://www.vapourbeauty.com

W3llPeople—http://www.w3llpeople.com

Weleda—http://www.weleda.com

Zuii Organics—http://www.zuiiorganic.com

Zuzu Luxe—http://www.gabrielcosmeticsinc.com/index.cfm/
category/3/zuzu-luxe.cfm

TOP PICKS

FACE • • • 3 POINTS

- 100% Pure Coffee Bean Eye Cream
- Dr. Hauschka Rose Day Cream
- Nude Skin Care Cleansing Facial Oil
- Yes To Carrots Lip Balm

HAIR • • • 3 POINTS

- Burt's Bees Grapefruit and Sugar Beet Shampoo
- Rene Furterer Natural Dry Shampoo
- Whole Foods 365 Shampoo and Conditioner
- Weleda Rosemary Hair Oil

BODY • • • 3 POINTS

- Burt's Bees Aloe & Witch Hazel Hand Sanitizer
- Duchess Marden Body Serum
- Farm Aesthetics Organic Bugscreen

- Galen Labs Lemon Eucalyptus & Tea Tree Dead Sea Bath Salt
- Pratima Rose Organic Bath Oil and Salts
- Ren Body Lotion
- Revolution Organics All Over Body Balm

USE GREEN MAKEUP • • • 3 POINTS

- Dr. Hauschka Illuminating Powder
- Jane Iredale Lip Gloss
- Revolution Organics Blush
- Well People Narcissist Stick Foundation
- Zuii Organics Eye Shadow
- ZuZu Luxe Mascara

USE DIY IDEAS • • • 3 POINTS

- *Olive oil* is a great natural moisturizer for your face.
- *Coconut oil* is a fantastic balm for your body.
- *Brown Sugar Body Scrub:* Mix ½ cup granulated brown sugar with 3 tablespoons almond oil and 10 drops vanilla essential oil. Scrub it on in the shower and rinse it off. Be careful with the bottoms of your feet; it can be slippery.
- *Avocado Mask:* Mash an avocado fully until creamy, then add 1 tablespoon raw honey and 1 tablespoon organic yogurt. Rub it on your face and let it sit for 15 minutes. Rinse and pat dry. This is a great mask for moisturizing, removing dead cells, and calming the skin.

SLIM MYTH:
With the right cream, diet, or procedure, you can get rid of cellulite.

FAST FACT: Sadly, there's absolutely nothing we can do about cellulite. I've tried pretty much everything and to no avail. Cellulite has more to do with the structure of your connective tissue than with your body fat percentage. That's why even slim people can get it. Many have theorized about why we get cellulite. Theories range from genetics to hormones, but the reality is that at the moment there's nothing we can do to make it better. Don't get sucked in by expensive creams or painful procedures; cellulite is one of those blights—you either get it or you don't. There's no really solid reason to date as to why, and no dependable solution to it.

- *Shea Butter Lip Balm:* You will need 1 teaspoon organic grated beeswax or beeswax pellets, 2½ teaspoons organic shea butter, 1 teaspoon organic sweet almond oil, 2 drops vitamin E oil, 2 drops organic tea tree oil, and 8 drops organic rose oil. Heat all the ingredients in a small saucepan over low heat, stir, and blend together. Pour into a small container and let cool. It makes a great gift.
- *Sea Salt Scrub:* Combine 1 cup Dead Sea salt, 15 drops essential lavender oil, and ¼ cup dried lavender. Store in a glass Mason jar. Scoop and use.
- *Cucumber Facial:* Simply cut two slices of cucumber and place them on your eyes. Cucumber nourishes, hydrates, and helps to reduce the appearance of dark circles.

DRUGS THAT SABOTAGE YOUR SLIM

CHECK OUT YOUR SCRIPS • • • 3 POINTS

About 70 percent of people in the United States are overweight, and in a cruel catch-22, many of the drugs used to treat obesity-linked conditions such as diabetes, high blood pressure, and depression can themselves cause weight gain. The following medications are known to contribute to obesity: Allegra, Deltasone (prednisone), Depakote, depot medroxyprogesterone acetate (DMPA), Diabinese, Endep, Elavil, Insulase, Paxil, Prozac, Remeron, Tenormin, Thorazine, Vanatrip, Zyprexa, and Zyrtec. Some pretty provocative research shows just how much havoc these drugs wreak when it comes to your weight. Before you decide to do anything about these meds, if you're on them or considering taking them, consult with your doctor.

Allergy Meds. A 2010 study at Yale University that was published in the journal *Obesity* found that individuals who take antihista-mines regularly (the primary drugs in question were both over-the-counter, Zyrtec and Allegra) are heavier than those who never take them. They also concluded that a person taking these drugs is *55 percent more likely to be overweight* than someone not taking them. Researchers can't yet confirm the exact relationship between the drugs and allergies, but other studies have shown that antihista-mines trigger an increase in appetite and have a sedating effect. Who wants to exercise when you're in the ozone and craving food? A 2006 survey of those who use oral corticosteroid drugs on a long-term basis (particularly the high doses needed in the treatment of asthma) indicated that 60 to 80 percent of those surveyed gained weight. The risk also seems to be higher when these drugs are taken orally than when breathed in through inhalants.

Antibiotics. Here's a good one. I've already suggested that you eat clean meat, without antibiotics and hormones. Doesn't it make sense that if livestock are being fed drugs to fatten them up, then maybe humans who consume drug-infused meat will get fat, too? Researchers are now thinking the same thing, examining the rela-tionship between antibiotics and obesity. They believe that these drugs may be impacting the bacteria in our gut and affecting our ability to metabolize nutrients, thus causing weight gain and meta-bolic syndrome. A recent study, published in *Nature,* shows a cor-relation between rising U.S. obesity rates and the use of antibiotics.

Antidepressants and mood stabilizers. Depakote is used to treat bipolar disorder and seizures and to prevent migraines. A 2007 study tracking epileptic patients taking Depakote found that 44 percent of the women and 24 percent of the men gained 11 pounds or more over the course of about a year. One of its known side affects is to increase appetite, causing weight gain. Lithium shows a similar weight-gain pattern, though with a fewer adverse effects than Depakote.

Zyprexa and Clozapine are antipsychotics, used to treat schizophrenia and bipolar disorder. A 2005 study indicated that 30 percent of individuals using Zyprexa put on 7 percent or more body weight within 18 months. Both drugs promote heavy-duty potent antihistamine activity and inhibit serotonin, which researchers theorize may trigger weight gain.

Elavil, Endep, and Vanatrip (amitriptyline) are TCAs, or tricyclic antidepressants. These drugs influence neurotransmitter and antihistamine activity, which in turn affects energy levels and appetite regulation (affecting serotonin, dopamine, and acetylcholine); they are the probable cause of related weight gain.

Insulin. This one is interesting and frankly seems a little backward: take a drug to control type 2 diabetes and get fat from it? A study found that individuals dependent on insulin gained an average of 11 pounds during their first three years on the drug. Half of the weight gain generally occurred in the first three months.

Beta blockers. Tenormin, Lopressor, and Inderal (propranolol) are used to control high blood pressure. These drugs are known to slow calorie-burning potential and cause fatigue, making it pretty difficult to seriously exercise and pretty easy to pack on the pounds. In a study, those taking Tenormin gained about 5 more pounds than did those in a placebo group in their first few months on the drug. While your blood pressure may stabilize, your weight may not.

Again, make sure to talk to your doctor about the side effects of any medication you're taking. If weight gain is one of them, ask if there's an alternative medication that doesn't produce this unwanted side effect. If not, ask if your doctor can wean you off the drug over time in tandem with your other lifestyle changes.

ADD IT UP, DROP IT OFF

GIVE YOURSELF 3 POINTS

☐ The center will increase your center.

☐ Keep your head down.

☐ Don't shop while you're hungry—*ever*!

☐ Be wholesome.

☐ Serve it up.

☐ Keep it short and simple.

☐ Check: one, two, three.

☐ Be a matchmaker.

☐ Say it loud.

☐ Get out your decoder ring.

☐ If it sounds too good . . .

☐ Be salt savvy.

☐ Be sugar savvy.

☐ Be like Grandma—get your fiber.

☐ Break the rules.

☐ Swap it out.

☐ Keep essentials on hand.

☐ Slip a disc.

☐ Use the clean hygiene, skin care, and beauty brands Paige loves.

☐ Face

☐ Hair

☐ Body

☐ Use green makeup.

☐ Use DIY ideas.

☐ Check out your scrips.

GIVE YOURSELF 2 POINTS

☐ Be like Santa.

☐ Go solo; don't take the kids.

☐ Go low.

☐ Make a clean cut.

☐ Spice it up.

☐ Start flashing.

☐ Dry off.

☐ Chill out and save calories.

☐ Keep it firm.

☐ Build a toolbox.

☐ Use green brands.

☐ Use homemade cleaning essentials.

GIVE YOURSELF 1 POINT

☐ Cart it around.

☐ Wear your skinny jeans.

☐ Go fish.

☐ Don't cut corners.

☐ Judge food by its cover.

☐ Exhaust the cashier.

☐ Kick the can.

☐ Chew mint gum.

☐ Add to your recipe deck.

☐ Grab a chair.

☐ If you build it, you'll use it.

_____ **Total *points* for Chapter 3**

_____ **Total number of *tips* I'm incorporating**

....

CHAPTER 4

ON THE GO

Now you know how to navigate taking nutrition and fitness into your own hands, and how to construct a home environment that will keep you healthy and slim. Next we need to address how to manage environments and circumstances where you can't control every aspect, so the outcome will still work out in your favor. This is the area where most people get lost.

I can't tell you how many people's weight-loss regimens have been ruined because they binge at a party, or don't know how to eat out properly, or don't get in their workouts while they're on the road, or suffer from a grueling work schedule, and so on.

This chapter tackles it all. It will give you everything you need to know so your exercise and diet regimen will be failsafe when you're away from home.

Party Time

We're going to start off with one of the most challenging "out and about" scenarios: eating healthy at a party. This one is tough; you don't want to be rude and tell the host what they should and shouldn't be serving. You can't really bring your own food, unless you're specifically asked to contribute a dish (more on that in a moment). What to do? Follow my lead, with these simple ways to stay on track while whoopin' it up.

SLIM CELEBRATING

FILL UP YOUR TANK • • • 3 POINTS

Eat before you hit the party. If you've eaten, you won't be tempted by foods that are less than healthy. If it's a dinner party where the sole purpose is to eat, you can still have a little snack before you go. Then if the food at the party isn't on your personal food list, you won't be hungry, so you can eat much less of it.

BE A GRACIOUS GUEST • • 2 POINTS

Bring a healthy dish for everyone to share. You'll be helping the hostess and being a considerate guest. Plus, you'll get to hide your secret agenda of bringing something slimming you can eat, if there's nothing else healthy there.

STAY AWAY FROM THE BUFFET • • • 3 POINTS

I can't understand why anyone who wants to lose weight would congregate by the buffet table—it's the ultimate diet danger zone. It's much easier to avoid mindless munching if you station yourself with your friends, and a plate, away from a laden table.

CHOOSE WISELY • • • 3 POINTS

At most parties you will find at least a couple of healthy, or healthier, choices to nosh on. Pass by the deep-fried junk and the pigs in a blanket and head for the veggie platter, shrimp plate, fruit platter, and cold cuts instead.

LIGHTEN UP • • 2 POINTS

If you're the host of the party, be responsible when deciding what food to serve. Pick the lighter options from among your party food favorites. Offer baked corn chips and salsa instead of Doritos and fattening cheese or bean dips. Go with baked chicken wings instead of fried. Use hummus instead of ranch dressing for your veggie sticks. Pick raw or dry roasted nuts instead of those salted and roasted in oil. Order a thin-crust veggie pizza with light cheese instead of the deep dish with the works on top. You follow me? Good. Now, go have some fun.

INDULGE RESPONSIBLY • • • 3 POINTS

You don't have to deprive yourself. If there's something that you really want to try, or you're just feeling left out of the festivities, you *can* have a treat. You just can't eat *full* servings of all the treats. Remember to follow the 80/20 rule and indulge appropriately. Fill up on healthy stuff, so that you'll be full when you get to the treat. You'll naturally eat less of it. Then pick one thing you want to indulge in and go for it.

SAMPLE SMALL PORTIONS • • • 3 POINTS

Use a small plate and *take a taste* of everything you want to try. That way you'll get to enjoy and participate fully in the party, but you won't get a ton of calories. In other words, undersize your portions, and you'll enjoy yourself as well as watch your waistline!

SIP FROM A WINEGLASS • 1 POINT

You can still be in party mode even when you aren't drinking. The entire time my partner Heidi was pregnant, she got all her beverages in a wineglass, so she felt like she was part of the festivities. Try some sparkling water with a splash of cranberry—it almost looks the part.

WATER BACK • 1 POINT

If you do want to drink, remember to slim your drinks as I mentioned in Chapter 1, then alternate every cocktail with a glass of water. This will help you hold your liquor, so you'll drink less, and it'll keep you from being ravenously hungry—a twofer if I do say so!

BE A PARTY PLANNER • • 2 POINTS

If you like to party hard, watch your daily calorie intake during the daytime, in the hours before a party. Don't skip meals—you'll be starving by the time you get to the event. Just choose your foods wisely all day and be calorie savvy. Eat a lettuce-wrapped sandwich or a salad with protein for lunch, to save calories for a party splurge later.

Restaurant Survival

The number-one way most of us sabotage our slim is by eating out. That's not to say you can't do it—before I had the kids, I did it seven nights a week. (I'm a terrible cook.) As in everything else, the key to success in eating out is *how* you do it. The following straight-forward, easy-to-follow guidelines will ensure that your hot body remains that way.

SLIM DINING

SIDESTEP IT • • • 3 POINTS

Get all sauces and dressings on the side so you can control the amount you put on top. Some salad dressings and condiments can add 100 or more calories in just a tablespoon. That's crazy. Try dipping your fork into the dressing and then into your salad for each bite. Or put a thin spread of the Thousand Island on your burger. You get the idea.

> **EZ CALORIE CUT**
> Instead of 5 ounces of alfredo sauce, have 7 ounces of marinara sauce. **CUT: 129 CALORIES**

SWAP SIDES • • • 3 POINTS

This one is so important. Sides can be a killer. A cheeseburger from a place like Johnny Rockets has around 500 calories, but when you add the fries and the drink, it gets up into the 1,000-calorie range. *Insane!* Or let's say you're being good about watching your calorie intake and order the halibut steak, but it comes with roasted pota-toes on the side. You start off just eating one but end up eating all. Your light dinner has just turned into 700-plus calories. Instead, always swap a starch for greens. Side salads (with dressing on the side, of course) and *steamed* veggies are the way to go.

JUMP THE GUN • • 2 POINTS

Prevent temptation by telling the waiter in advance that you want no bread or chips, before they hit the table. People say will-

SLIM MYTH:

Raw vegetables are healthier than cooked.

FAST FACT: Raw food fanatics constantly claim that vegetables lose critical nutrients when they're cooked. The truth is that while cooking veggies can potentially destroy some of their vitamin C content, it can have the opposite effect on many other vitamins. For example, cooking tomatoes boosts their amount of lycopene. (Cook them with a little olive oil, and your body's ability to absorb the lycopene just went up, too.) According to *Scientific American,* cooked carrots, spinach, mushrooms, asparagus, cabbage, peppers, and other vegetables also contain more antioxidants, like carotenoids and ferulic acid, than their raw equivalents.

Some argue that raw veggies have more enzymes than cooked, but registered dietitians tell us that while heating food above 118 degrees can deactivate certain plant enzymes, those enzymes are made to support the survival of plants; they're not essential to human health. Our bodies are actually very efficient in producing enzymes. Plus, plant enzymes are generally inactive by the time they reach our digestive tract, regardless of whether we've eaten the veggie raw or cooked.

Last, many people have a hard time breaking down raw vegetables in their gastrointestinal tract; hence Beano was created and has become so successful. Lightly cooking vegetables helps to break down the plants' cell walls (fibers called cellulose), making them easier to digest. Regardless of whether you eat them raw or cooked, there is one indisputable fact: we should all get more veggies in our diets.

power is like a muscle. It's true—if you constantly expose it to temptation, it gets fatigued. Don't needlessly put yourself in harm's way. Safeguard your health by removing trouble before it comes near you.

BE HIGH-MAINTENANCE ••• 3 POINTS

Customize your order to avoid excess calories. Ask the waiter to tell the kitchen to grill the fish, not sauté it, or to put the burger on lettuce leaves instead of a bun, or to scrape the excess bread out of the inside of your bagel. I know many of you will have issues with doing this. You feel bad asking a chef to go out of his or her way, or you think you're inconveniencing the waiter. Nonsense. It's your money, and you have every right to get what you want and need. Trust me when I tell you that restaurants are used to it and will think nothing of it. Plus, they know there are thousands of eateries where you could have gone to spend your hard-earned cash, so it's truly a privilege that you chose their establishment over another place to eat. Ultimately, even if I'm wrong (which I'm not), the worst that can happen is they say no. Then you leave or make a note not to go back there.

FIB • 1 POINT

I hate giving you this tip because I always want you to be decent and live in truth, but learning how to assert yourself doesn't happen overnight. If you're still embarrassed to ask for special treatment, or too uncomfortable to ask for what you need, tell a white lie: say you're allergic. I know it's controversial to suggest this, but women in particular can really have trouble standing up for their own needs and wants. So if you want the broccoli soup puréed without cream, tell the waiter you're lactose intolerant. You can do this with just about anything you don't want on or in your food. If you don't want croutons or a bun on your burger, tell them you have a gluten intolerance. I know it's a crazy thing to say, but it doesn't hurt anyone. And if it saves your health and prevents you from developing a muffin top, who really cares?

BE CREATIVE • 1 POINT

Order without looking at the menu. Almost every restaurant in the world has the basics—veggies, grains, and protein. If you go in knowing what you want, I guarantee you'll be able to make a meal. Even at some of the most fattening food chains, I've been able to stay on my regimen by ordering fish, chicken, or steak grilled, baked, or broiled with a side salad, or veggies and steamed brown rice. In a way this goes back to the "Be high-

maintenance" tip. Tell the waiter what you want to eat and how you want to eat it. You're a paying customer. The restaurant should be happy to oblige.

PICK YOUR BATTLES • • 2 POINTS

Find a group of restaurants you like, and make them your go-to spots. This way you build an arsenal of places where you know there'll be healthy things to eat. I have five places I rotate out for lunch, and maybe five places for when we bring food in. I know I can trust them all to provide healthy dishes that'll keep me on the slim path. Look for places that list the calorie info on the menu—most states these days actually require it. Le Pain Quotidien does this, as does Chipotle, Applebee's, Chili's, Olive Garden, and Red Lobster. I hope you don't end up at some of these obscenely fattening restaurant chains, but if you live in a place with limited options, at least you'll know how to make the slimmest choice by looking at the calorie counts on the menu. And make the restaurants you choose accommodate you, so that you can be high-maintenance, as previously discussed.

BE SOUP SMART • • 2 POINTS

You're always going to need to make choices, and some are smarter than others. If you're a soup person, be sure to opt for broth-based soups like purées, minestrone, and chicken soup instead of cream-based ones like clam chowder or cream of anything. If you're confused about whether the soup has cream in it, just ask. Many veggie soups can go both ways. Some are purées, which are great options, but some have cream, oil, or butter added to them. When in doubt, ask your server.

DON'T FORGET TO DRY OFF •• 2 POINTS

Always ask for your food to be cooked dry. This simply means using little or no butter or oil. You want your eggs scrambled dry. You want your toast, waffles, or pancakes dry, meaning no butter on top. Pretty much anything that's cooked in oil or butter can be made with minimal "grease." You just have to ask.

GET IT TO GO •• 2 POINTS

God bless America and her massive portions. You might think you're getting your money's worth, as the waiter sets that Italian dinner plate down in front of you, but what you've really bought yourself is a vat of pasta with a side of cellulite, saddlebags, and maybe even a heart attack. Yay? If you're like me, you might have issues about "wasting" food when you don't clean your plate. Instead of trying to talk you out of this backward psychology, I'm going to tell you about a really easy way to work with it: before your waiter brings the dish to the table, ask him or her to wrap half of it up in a to-go box. This way you'll have two meals for the price of one, and only half the calories, and you won't feel like you're cheating the kids that are starving in Africa. Hate to say it, but I still feel that way. Oy.

BE GENEROUS •• 2 POINTS

Another option to manage the massive portion dilemma is to share your entrée with your dining buddy. This idea rocks for two reasons: you not only will save on your calories, but you'll also save some cash by not purchasing that second entrée.

TAKE A PASS •• 2 POINTS

We get caught up in food rituals. Who says you have to order an appetizer plus an entrée and a dessert? Who really needs three courses of food? It's nuts. Skip the appetizer and go straight to the entrée. Again, you'll save some dough, and you'll save your physique. If it's a tradition you just must uphold, then ask for salad as your appetizer, without all the rich embellishments, and dressing on the side. Or have two appetizers for your main dish. If you feel the need to order courses, just choose smartly.

> **EZ CALORIE CUT**
> For an order of fried calamari, substitute 3 ounces of grilled calamari. **CUT: 812 CALORIES**

AVOID DANGER ••• 3 POINTS

This tip applies to everything in life, but for the purpose of this book, I want you to specifically avoid foods that are described by what I call "danger words": *smothered, loaded, tender, deep-fried,* and *creamy*. These words scream "I'm loaded with ridiculous amounts of calories. I'll wreck your diet. I'll make you feel sluggish and gross." When you see these words, avoid the dish at all costs. Unless, of course, you apply my "Be high-maintenance" tip and have them make it to your healthy specifics. If you do that, the dish will be a lot healthier and often unrecognizable to its original form. Danger removed.

PAT IT DOWN •• 2 POINTS

Have you ever gotten an omelet or a piece of pizza where the grease is pooling on top of it? Should you end up eating such an Item from time to time, ahem, it's easy to dab off the excess oil with a paper napkin to avoid adding insult to injury. You'd be amazed how many calories you can save by doing this, anywhere from 100 to 200 per pat-down.

SLIM MYTH:

Fat makes you fat.

FAST FACT: By this point in the book, I'm sure you've started to get it: fat doesn't make you fat; excess calories make you fat. Fats, just like healthy carbs and proteins, are essential for health. They support the cardiovascular, reproductive, immune, and nervous systems. They also help with maintaining a lean body and assist with consistent fat burning. That's right—eating fat burns fat! The chief function of essential fatty acids is the production of prostaglandins, which control functions like blood clotting, fertility, heart rate, and blood pressure. They also help immune function by regulating inflammation, thus assisting the body to fight infection. The only fly in this ointment is trans fats. They should be avoided at all costs.

BE MULTICULTURALLY SELECTIVE • • • 3 POINTS

When eating ethnic cuisine, look for the healthiest, slimmest options possible. Here are my top suggestions:

- Mexican. Choose grilled tacos in corn tortillas (only one tortilla per taco, please), or better yet, ask for a taco or burrito bowl (with salad instead of rice and no tortilla). Try carne asada, fajitas (ask for them dry or using little oil), and tostadas (don't eat the fried shell). For sides, have black beans (provided they aren't refried with lard).

> **EZ CALORIE CUT**
> Eating Mexican? Eliminate one tortilla from each soft taco—they usually come prepared with two, sometimes three.
> **CUT: 100 CALORIES EACH TACO**

- Greek. Pick souvlaki, kebabs, Greek salad, tabbouleh, hummus, yogurt, or pita bread.
- Asian. Try sashimi; seaweed salad; a chicken, shrimp, or beef satay (go easy on the peanut sauce); and brown rice. Get dishes steamed instead of sautéed, like shrimp with vegetables, paper-wrapped chicken, or moo goo gai pan.
- Indian. Enjoy tandoori, lentil-based soups, vindaloos, or vegetable dishes like *saag* prepared with little oil.

- Italian. Eat any grilled chicken or seafood selection, pasta primavera (without cream), or minestrone soup.

....

At Work

Another area of common concern and confusion that can sabotage your sexy, slim body is what to eat—and how to fit in exercise—when you're at work or struggling with a crazy work schedule. So many people are slaves to the nine-to-five grind. They're either chained to their desks or constantly on the run or on the road for work. All are murder to a healthy lifestyle. I understand this, believe me, and I've suffered from it personally. That's why I developed my own strategies to acquire and maintain slimness, while still achieving professional success. If your work has ever interfered with your workouts or your healthy eating habits, never fear. The advice that follows will help you find balance and get you as close as possible to "having it all."

EATS AT THE OFFICE

KEEP A PRIVATE STASH • • • 3 POINTS

I had a desk job for three years in my mid-twenties. I was a rat on a wheel working from eight to eight, trying to "keep up with the Joneses." After months of eating chips and soda from the vending machine, leftover crap from office meetings, and takeout food like pizza from the delivery place where all the other assistants ordered, I gained 5 pounds. That may not sound like a lot to you, but honestly, for my frame it was. It was also enough to make me feel uncomfortable. I wised up. I got a small, used mini-fridge and tucked it under my desk in my cubicle. That way I was able to stock up on my own healthy food. Guess what? The 5 extra pounds fell right off.

SEND A JIBJAB • 1 POINT

I can't tell you how many times I've seen the cake or cupcakes roll out for a coworker's birthday. Depending on the size of your office, these festivities can lead to calorie-blowing disaster—you can wind up indulging in birthday cake multiple times a week. After all, you don't want to be rude right? You don't want to waste food, right? Wrong! Send a happy birthday e-mail. Explain that you won't be making it over for the celebration because you're "saving the extra calories" and can't handle the temptation. Let them know you love them and hope they have a rad birthday. End of story. I promise they'll understand. If they don't, forget them. They aren't really a friend if they can't support you in this.

Your only alternative is to campaign to switch the whole office over to a healthier alternative like frozen yogurt or fruit plates. Good luck with that. I tried it personally and didn't get very far. Why rain on the birthday person's parade? Just send an e-mail or stop by before the cake to offer your birthday wishes.

START A BANDWAGON ••• 3 POINTS

Communicate with your coworkers that you're on a health kick. See who you can get on board. Try to switch the TGIF happy hour ritual for a late-afternoon company basketball game. Or start a walking group before or after work, maybe even during lunch hour. Talk to your HR department about the food provided in morning meetings. Instead of bagels, bacon and cheese omelets, and muffins, plead your "slim" argument and get them to switch over to 100 percent whole-grain Ezekiel muffins, fruit plates, organic Greek yogurt, 100 percent whole-grain toast with scrambled eggs, and nitrate-free turkey bacon. And if HR doesn't agree to substitute all of these, see where they will compromise, and at least try to influence them to serve *something* healthy.

HAVE A PLAN • • • 3 POINTS

Sometimes temptation can't be avoided, but knowing it's coming ahead of time allows you to plan an effective strategy and a successful outcome. Here are the key danger zones you'll likely encounter and tactics for managing them.

1. If you're forced at some point to eat from a vending machine, choose yogurt, nuts and seeds, granola bars, mini pretzels, or string cheese. AVOID chips, cookies, pastries, candy bars, and soda.

2. At the morning meeting, if you're lucky and have healthy options, go with fruit, yogurt, half a low-fat bran muffin, oatmeal, dry toast, or eggs. AVOID bacon, pastries, bagels, jams, and cream cheese. If healthy options are never available, eat before you get to work, or bag your own healthy breakfast so you can eat with everyone else.

3. When your coworkers order takeout, choose the healthiest option possible from the menu. (Refer back to the "Be multiculturally selective" tip on page 120 if you need to.) If they're ordering Chinese, select the paper-wrapped chicken; if it's Italian, get a salad. (Even pizza joints have some kind of antipasto or salad—but skip the added meats and cheeses.) If they're ordering from a sandwich place, order a grilled chicken sandwich with lettuce, tomato, and mustard. Got it?

4. Combat a coworker's candy bowl by putting a fruit bowl on your desk. Try having healthier options in sight and within reach to help defend against temptation.

PACK IT IN • • • 3 POINTS

Just as your mom did when she sent you to school, you should pack and bring your lunch. Bringing healthy snacks to the office is great, but bringing healthy meals makes a huge difference. Spend one night each week cooking food that you can throw into a glass container. Then store it in the office fridge or your mini-fridge (the one you're going to purchase and stash under your desk if the company allows it). If cooking seems overwhelming or impossible to you, the other option is to bring healthy frozen foods to work. Although I'm not a fan, as most frozen foods are crap and filled with chemicals and preservatives, there are a few options out there that will suffice.

Look for these frozen-food brands: Amy's Organic, Healthy Choice 100% Natural (while not organic, it's free of artificial flavors, preservatives, and colors, making it a better option than most), Nature's Path, Cedar Lane, Trader Joe's, and 365 Organic.

SLIM MYTH:
Microwaving zaps the nutrients in food.

FAST FACT: What affects the nutrients in food is the level of heat and the amount of time you're cooking it, not the cooking method itself. The longer and hotter you cook a food, the more of certain heat- and water-sensitive nutrients you'll lose, especially vitamin C and thiamine (a B vitamin). The key is to cook your food lightly. Ironically, because microwave cooking often cooks foods more quickly, it can actually help to minimize nutrient losses.

COP A SQUAT • 1 POINT

Remember that scene from the movie *Pretty Woman* where Julia Roberts takes Richard Gere to the park for lunch to "cop a squat"? Grab a park bench or a spot in the grass and enjoy your lunch. The point is to eat away from your desk. One of the worst eating mistakes is to place yourself in an atmosphere where you can be easily distracted from the food in front of you. Remember our "Make it a production" tip on page 27? Eating in front of your computer is like eating in front of your television—bad.

Although you may think it's convenient or shows company loyalty to work through your lunch break, don't do it. Studies show that people who eat when they're distracted tend to overeat. Instead, stop and focus on the food. Not only will you eat less, you'll enjoy your food more. Maybe you'll even get a few moments out of your day to enjoy nature or the company of good friends, or to destress.

PLAY THE FIELD ● ● 2 POINTS

Suss out restaurants with healthy takeout menus that are close to your workplace. Keep a notebook listing them and stash it somewhere so that it's readily available. When it's time to eat, you and your coworkers are already set up for success, and you can choose a place you've already preapproved.

> **EZ CALORIE CUT**
> For a chicken burrito, substitute 3 soft chicken tacos. **CUT: 460 CALORIES**

GETTING EXERCISE IN ON THE JOB

I don't expect you to be busting out circuits while you're wearing your power suit, but there are plenty of ways to get in a bit of physical activity even in the midst of a hectic workday.

BE COMPETITIVE ● 1 POINT

Competition is a great incentive when it comes to workouts. I can't begin to tell you how many people have come up to me and told me they started a weight-loss competition at their office, and that they'd already lost x amount of pounds themselves and so had others. This is a great thing to initiate at work because it builds motivation, support, and camaraderie among coworkers. Get as many people on board as possible, and break the office up into weight-loss teams. Then try to structure team workouts with coworkers around the competition, like a yoga class before the morning meeting or a running group after work. Fostering such competition will not only champion your healthy lifestyle stand at the office, it will create a happier, healthier environment for all involved.

WALK 'N' TALK • • • 3 POINTS

Stand up and walk for the duration of your phone calls. If you're in a small cube, step side to side, do small knee lifts, or stretch while you talk. You'll burn 2 to 4 calories a minute. It adds up, really: you can burn 60 to 120 calories on a 30-minute phone call.

LOOK RIDICULOUS • • 2 POINTS

Sorry, I know the advice that I'm about to impart isn't necessarily advice you want to hear or adhere to, but it's important that you do it. I always felt ridiculous following it, but I did it anyway because I cared about the size of my ass more than I cared about what people at work thought of me. The advice is: do body-weight exercises at your desk. Try doing push-ups on the edge of the desk, squats (touch

---

BE NEAT AT WORK

- Park your car at the back of the lot.
- Leave the building and enjoy walking to meetings with coworkers.
- Get off the bus a few stops earlier.
- Hoof it to work.
- Ditch the elevator and take the stairs every chance you get.
- Deliver messages in person rather than by e-mail.
- Empty your own trash!

your bum to the seat of your chair for every rep), calf raises, lunges, and dips on your chair. I knocked out a set of these every hour or so. Take care of you—there's nothing silly about that.

PLAY BALL GAMES • 1 POINT

Sit on a stability ball instead of a chair to strengthen your abs and back and to improve posture. Sitting on a ball challenges your core all day long. Do ball bounces and seated ball jacks to increase circulation and to turn on your brain. Finally, use the ball to get in a few crunches, squats, and push-ups during a break before you head home.

GEAR UP •• 2 POINTS

Designate one of your file cabinets, or even just a corner of your cube, as an exercise locker. Seriously. I want you to store a pair of athletic shoes so you can use your breaks to take a quick, brisk walk or go for an even longer one during lunch. Stash a resistance tube so you can create a minicircuit of resistance training in your cube or office; let it double as a stretching tool to relieve muscles tired from sitting. Squeeze in a quick set between phone calls or meetings. Store some hand weights, too. Your back and upper body will thank you for it.

RRRRRING! ••• 3 POINTS

Set an alarm on your watch, phone, or computer to remind you to get up and move every hour.

HAVE COFFEE TO GO •• 2 POINTS

Get active on your coffee break. Change into walking shoes and zoom past the coffee machine and the coffee klatch in the lunchroom. (Of course, you can always invite them to join you.) Then log in a half mile or a full mile (inside or outside the building); it takes 10 minutes to walk a half mile, about 20 for a full. How long you walk depends on how much time you have for your break. On your way back in, grab your coffee and trot back to your work-station. It's a win-win in my opinion: some exercise and a quick caffeine fix.

....

Travel Secrets

This next section applies—as you may have guessed—to all things travel-related. Whether you're hauling yourself from place to place for work or are off having a luxurious vacation, any time you're on the road, you lose a little of the control and support that you now have at home. Try these tricks to stay on track.

EATS ON THE ROAD

STOCK UP •• 2 POINTS

Use your hotel room's minibar to stock healthy food from a local grocery store. I always do this when I travel to remote locations that have nothing but fast-food joints and gas stations on every corner. It may not be the most convenient thing to do, but it'll save your ass—literally.

BE RESOURCEFUL •• 2 POINTS

You know those little motels and hotels that don't have room ser-vice but always serve complimentary juice, Danish, and coffee in the morning? I can't tell you how many times I've been in places like this while traveling for work and felt like I had no options. Well, I came up with a solution! Bring oatmeal packets with you. Nature's Path Hemp Plus is my personal favorite. Then use the coffee maker in your room to make the hot water for it. Or pack a BPA-free

BlenderBottle with a wire mixer ball—it's light and compact. Use it to make a protein shake, or let it do double duty to hold water so you stay hydrated.

GRAB AND GO • • • 3 POINTS

Grab your favorite snacks that pack well and bring them with you. I always bring protein powder and oatmeal packets, as I mentioned, but I also take 22 Days protein bars, Kind bars, Justin's peanut butter packets, whole-grain crackers, dry roasted nuts, organic turkey or beef jerky, freeze-dried fruit (different from dried fruit, it's lower in calories and has less sugar). This should cover you in a pinch and help you navigate the airport when healthy options are scarce and you can't get a real meal. Plus, all these items are approved for carry-on. Meals on planes are nonexistent these days in coach—but you can toss these snacks in your bag and rest easy.

MAKE CONVENIENCE COUNT
• • 2 POINTS

Have you heard the term *food desert*? It means a place where there are no healthy food options for ten-plus miles in every direction, and there's just a wasteland of gas stations and fast-food joints. Occasionally, you'll have to travel to one, and sometimes when you're on the road, you'll find only gas stations and convenience stores. Should this be the case, here are the go-to options you can almost always find at any mini-mart, even in no-man's-land: hard-boiled eggs, cheese sticks, yogurt, popchips, protein bars, nuts, fruit, and the healthiest cereal option available.

SLIM MYTH:
You should go number two after every meal, or your metabolism isn't functioning properly.
FAST FACT: A healthy, slim person may not move their bowels after every meal, let alone three times a day. Constipation or irregular bowel is defined as having fewer than three stools per week. Therefore you may be more normal than you think. If you feel you're getting stopped up, drink water, eat whole grains, add some flaxseed to your cereal or yogurt, and eat plenty of high-fiber veggies. When in doubt, you can always try prunes—they work too!

CHOOSE THE LEAST OF ALL EVILS •• 2 POINTS

God help me for having to write this, but if you're forced to go to a fast-food place, under duress or threat of bodily harm by a desperate friend (let me pretend, please, that there would be no other reason for you to find yourself there), look for a Starbucks, Chipotle, Baja Fresh, El Pollo Loco, Au Bon Pain, or Subway. These places at least have sandwiches that don't contain thousands of calories, and they provide healthier options like grilled fish tacos and salads. (Just remember to get all condiments and dressings on the side!) When I'm in this position, I'll get the six-inch veggie from Subway, no cheese or mayo, and add in avocado. (And I have them scrape the excess bread from inside the sandwich roll.)

> **EZ CALORIE CUT**
> In your sandwich, replace 1 ounce of whole-fat cheese with 1 ounce (1 slice) of low-fat cheese.
> **CUT: 56 CALORIES**

FITNESS ON THE FLY

ENGAGE IN AIRPORT EXERCISE • 1 POINT

Don't want to skip your workout? Want to make every minute of your trip count? Whether you're a workaholic road warrior who spends half your life in airports, or you're stuck on a stopover en route to a villa vacation, you can grab a workout before you even take off. A cool website, www.airportgyms.com, offers a unique service: it posts listings of airport gyms, airport exercise clubs, and fitness centers within a short distance of airports in and around major U.S. and Canadian cities. You can even check out the nearest gym online to see what it offers, so you're geared up and ready to exercise when you get there.

FLY FIT • 1 POINT

One of the worst things you can do to your body is sit for hours on a flight and never get up from your seat. If you're flying for more than an hour, it's easy to feel just as stiff and cramped as you do at work if you sit all day. Not moving around for long periods of time can cause problems with circulation. For anyone who has existing circulatory issues, it's even more important to move about the cabin when you can, to prevent blood clots from forming.

Here are some ways to get your move on in a plane:

- Avoid crossing your legs or ankles for long periods of time. Curl and uncurl your toes. Pull one knee at a time up toward your chest. Stretch your back, rounding your spine forward and arching it back.
- March in place, lifting your knees. I know this looks silly, but you'll feel much better than the people sitting next to you do.
- If you're not completely squashed like a sardine and have a little room, bend forward, reach for your feet, and hang like a rag doll.
- Stretch your arms overhead, grasp your opposite wrist, and stretch, then do the other side.
- Simulate biceps curls using your water bottle. Press up for modified triceps dips by pushing down on the seat arms.
- Twist and stretch your torso, placing your opposite hand on the seat arm and looking behind you. Repeat in the other direction.
- Try to stand up every hour you're in the air. Before you head back to your seat, stop at the back of the plane and do push-ups on the wall. (It's great for conversations, trust me.)
- Do deep yogic (belly) breathing. Inhale through your nose, expanding your belly, and slowly exhale through your nose. Not only is this great for calming nerves, it helps to balance

the left and right sides of your brain and circulate oxygen throughout your body. On a plane it's particularly great to do because your circulation is already compromised.

BE PICKY •• 2 POINTS

Stay at a hotel with a gym. If that's not an option, stay at a place with a gym nearby so you can get a guest pass. Most big chain gyms offer a free weekly pass on their websites as incentives to join—download it and save the gym fee. Another thing to consider: if and when you join a gym at home, look for a chain that's as national as possible, and sign up for all clubs. I do this with Crunch. That way I can work out at any Crunch gym when I travel. While they aren't in all parts of the country, I'm covered when I'm in California, Florida, and New York.

BE ACTION PACKED ••• 3 POINTS

Bring a fitness DVD, pop it in your computer, and get your move on. Or bring a resistance tube—it's cheap and portable. Toss it around the leg of the bed and get in your chest flys, military presses, rows, curls—you can add resistance to just about any exercise with this tubing. You can also use an app on your phone. My Slim-Down Solution app has tons of exercises with demonstrations available.

PLAY CARDS •• 2 POINTS

One warning before you read on—this one was introduced to me by Bob Harper. At the airport's convenience store, grab a deck of playing cards. Not only can they keep you entertained on your flight, they can give you a sinister workout in your hotel room. The first step is to assign an exercise to each suit. Say burpees for spades, push-ups for diamonds, sit-ups for clubs, and squats for hearts. Then go through the entire deck of cards and do the assigned number of exercises per card. So a 4 of clubs would mean you do 4 sit-ups, an 8 of spades would mean 8 burpees. Assign the face cards a value of 10, and the ace is 11. (No, it's not a 1—this is not blackjack, and it's not optional.) Try to keep it moving, and rest as little as possible. I promise you'll get an insane workout at little cost within a minimal space.

BE DEMANDING •• 2 POINTS

Check and see if the hotel TV's On Demand programming offers free workouts. Also, see if the hotel has simple equipment—a yoga mat, pair of dumbbells, or the like—that you can take back to your room.

HAVE AN ADVENTURE •• 2 POINTS

If you're on holiday, plan an active vacation, and try fitness regimens that are new to you. Go paddleboarding in Hawaii. Mountain-bike in Moab. Hike the Grand Canyon. River-raft or kayak the Kern River. Snowboard or ski in Sun Valley or Aspen. By making fitness part of your vacation lifestyle, you'll expose yourself to new things and prevent yourself from packing on pounds when packing your bags.

SIGHTSEE •• 2 POINTS

Walk the town. Often when I've gone on what should be the most fattening vacations (hello, Paris food fest!), I've actually come home a pound or two lighter. That's because I spent all day on my feet sightseeing. Get out, meet the people, take in some history, and see the place! Being on your feet for hours at a time, even when you aren't "exercising hard," will burn lons of calories and also allow you to take in some culture.

> **SLIM MYTH:**
> **Sweating eliminates toxins.**
> **FAST FACT:** Only 1 percent of the toxins that leave our bodies are excreted through our sweat glands. The main role of sweating is to regulate our body temperature; it's our natural cooling system. The main organs responsible for excreting waste are actually the gastrointestinal tract, liver, kidneys, immune system, and lungs.

GET WET •• 2 POINTS

I can't tell you how many vacations I take where I get my workout in the pool. This is a big one for people with kids. My kids love the pool, and I play with them or swim laps while they play. It's a great fitness resource, if weather permits, for hard-core workouts or active fun family time.

HAPPY TRAILS TO YOU ·· 2 POINTS

Ask the hotel staff or search the Web for local parks, hiking paths, and jogging routes. You can also take matters into your own hands by checking out www.trails.com. This website offers great options and resources for practically anywhere in the world you might find yourself.

ADD IT UP, DROP IT OFF

GIVE YOURSELF 3 POINTS

- ☐ Fill up your tank.
- ☐ Stay away from the buffet.
- ☐ Choose wisely.
- ☐ Indulge responsibly.
- ☐ Sample small portions.
- ☐ Sidestep it.
- ☐ Swap sides.
- ☐ Be high-maintenance.
- ☐ Avoid danger.
- ☐ Be multiculturally selective.
- ☐ Keep a private stash.
- ☐ Start a bandwagon.
- ☐ Have a plan.
- ☐ Pack it in.
- ☐ Walk 'n' talk.
- ☐ Rrrrring!
- ☐ Grab and go.
- ☐ Be action packed.

GIVE YOURSELF 2 POINTS

- ☐ Be a gracious guest.
- ☐ Lighten up.
- ☐ Be a party planner.
- ☐ Jump the gun.
- ☐ Pick your battles.
- ☐ Be soup smart.
- ☐ Don't forget to dry off.

☐ Get it to go.

☐ Be generous.

☐ Take a pass.

☐ Pat it down.

☐ Play the field.

☐ Look ridiculous.

☐ Gear up.

☐ Have coffee to go.

☐ Stock up.

☐ Be resourceful.

☐ Make convenience count.

☐ Choose the least of all evils.

☐ Be picky.

☐ Play cards.

☐ Be demanding.

☐ Have an adventure.

☐ Sightsee.

☐ Get wet.

☐ Happy trails to you.

GIVE YOURSELF 1 POINT

☐ Sip from a wineglass.

☐ Water back.

☐ Fib.

☐ Be creative.

☐ Send a Jibjab.

☐ Cop a squat.

☐ Be competitive.

☐ Play ball games.

☐ Engage in airport exercise.

☐ Fly fit.

_____ **Total *points* for Chapter 4**

_____ **Total number of *tips* I'm incorporating**

CHAPTER 5

STAYING MOTIVATED

This chapter may not seem critical, as it doesn't directly pertain to weight loss, *but* it is, and here's why. I can give you all the info. I can make it easy to apply and affordable. I can spoon-feed it to you and hold your hand while you digest it. But if you aren't motivated to utilize it and make it your way of life, then none of what I've brought you in these pages matters. I've basically wasted my time writing this book, and you've wasted your money buying it and your time reading it. As if this thought weren't annoying enough, think about what's really at stake here—your health, your confidence, your quality of life, your relationships, your sex drive, and (insert practically everything awesome here). All of these are negatively affected when your weight and health aren't optimal.

Not living up to your potential or living the life you deserve is a damn shame. I want you to have everything you want for yourself. Honestly, you deserve it. We all do. But staying on track doesn't come without some effort—you know that. You can trust that the guidance and instruction outlined in this chapter will make the work far more palatable and possibly even enjoyable.

Motivate, Inspire, and Incentivize

ATTITUDE ADJUSTMENT

MAKE IT PERSONAL • • • 3 POINTS

Before you take that first step on the treadmill or steam your first piece of broccoli, I want you to make a Slim List. It's supersimple to do and will tell you a lot about yourself. Don't worry, it'll be fun. Write down all the reasons you want to be healthy, and how you think being slim will improve your life.

Many people, when searching for motivation, look outward, and while that can help to catalyze an initial change, lasting motivation must come from within. As I've said, leading the slim life isn't always easy. Although I've tried to make it as uncomplicated and stress-free as possible for you, ultimately there'll be some sacrifice involved. Sacrifice is part of being a grown-up, isn't it? To help you manage this fact of life, you have to find your "why." Why is the sacrifice worth it—to *you*? There's a famous quote from Nietzsche that goes something like this: "If you have a *why* to live for, you can tolerate any *how*."

Identify your *why*. Why is staying motivated important to you? Be specific. Make it very personal and detailed. Don't just say things like "I want to be healthy." What does that mean? What would that look like in your life? Do you want to play hockey with your kids? Look amazing at spring break? Wear high-fashion clothes? Live to be one hundred? Make your baby daddy sorry he left you for the secretary? Have sex with the lights on? Whatever your motives, write them down and post that list everywhere you can. Let your wants, your needs, and your desires motivate you!

....

SLIM MYTH:

If you lose weight too fast, you won't keep it off.

FAST FACT: Ridiculous. I've taken 100 pounds off of a man in 6 weeks, and 3 years later he's still proving my point. It's not the speed with which you take the weight off that matters—it's the method by which you did it. And a recent study conducted at the University of Florida also proves my point: it revealed that losing weight quickly in the early stages of a weight-loss program may be more beneficial, over the long term, both for losing the weight and for keeping it off. The researchers indicated that those who lost weight quickly were five times more likely to achieve clinically significant weight loss by an 18-month marker than those who lost weight at a slower rate. As long as you do it through exercise and clean eating, as opposed to starvation, there's no reason for you to put the weight back on, other than unresolved emotional issues or struggles.

....

ESTABLISH YOUR AGENDA • • • 3 POINTS

Once you've established why you want to get healthy, the next step is to figure out how you're going to do it. This is where setting goals comes in to play. People always talk about how important it is to have a goal and "write it down." That's very broad, vague advice and likely why most don't achieve the goals they set. One key to setting a useful and achievable goal is to create it using a few important guidelines:

- **Make your goal realistic.** Your ultimate goal must be truly attainable. If you work all the time and have a family to take care of, you won't be able to lose 100 pounds in 3 months, or even 20 pounds in 1 month. It's just not a workable possibility for you given your other commitments. You can still lose weight, however. Take a look at your life, and figure out what is a realistic amount of time you can commit to your exercise regimen, and then set the target where you can hit it. Under the scenario above, I'd say 20 pounds in 3 months is an ambitious goal that won't overwhelm you.

- **Make it measurable.** Don't say something like "I want to be thin and healthy." My *Biggest Loser* contestants say that all the time. But when I ask them what that actually means in real terms, they have no answer. If you don't have a clear idea of what something looks like, how will you ever achieve it? Instead, try saying "I want my blood pressure at 120/80." Or "I want to be able to run a half-marathon." Or "I want to lose 60 pounds."

BEHOLD THE POWER OF THE PYRAMID • • • 3 POINTS

Once your long-term goal is established, it can be pretty overwhelming, and many people struggle to keep sight of the big picture. It's easy to become intimidated when you think of everything you'll have to do to get to where you ultimately want to be. The trick is to realize that achieving a long-term goal must be done by meeting a series of short-term goals that are not just about the outcome but about the process of getting there. You must plot and plan how you're going to achieve the long-term goal in manageable stages. One of the best ways to do this is to create a goal pyramid that breaks the big goal into small, attainable short-term goals. This will allow you to literally plot a course of action, something that connects the things you're doing at this moment to the future you envision for yourself. Put your ultimate goal right at the top of the pyramid, then follow it underneath with monthly, weekly, daily, and immediate goals. For example:

Ultimate goal: I want to lose 25 pounds in 3 months.

Monthly goals: Each month I will drop 8 pounds.

Weekly goals: Each week I will lose 2 pounds. I will get to the gym 4 times this week. I will create a calorie deficit of 1,000 calories a day.

Daily goals: I will call my friend to switch carpool days so I can hit that boot camp class on Wednesdays and Fridays. I will make healthy food for the rest of the week so I'm able to hit my set calorie deficit. I will do research on restaurants in the area where I can get slimming meals. I will buy a Body Media Armband so I can track the calories I burn.

You see, using this formula you can break that long-term goal into a manageable action plan or road map that will lead you straight to your desired destination.

PAINT A PICTURE • • • 3 POINTS

Don't worry if you can't draw. I'm talking about a mental picture. Visualize yourself at the precipice of your goal; then see yourself achieving it. Creative visualization uses the power of the mind to inspire us and create the outcomes we want. Visions of achievement help you believe in your potential to turn your dreams into your reality. Picturing what you want and how you want to get it is a cornerstone to the process of making your dreams come true.

There are several important components to using this tool effectively:

- **Be specific.** If you want to be healthy, create a vision of *exactly* what healthy looks like. What clothes are you wearing? What activities are you doing with your strong, slim body? Are you running a 5K, playing with your kids, dancing with your significant other, or walking your daughter down the aisle? The more details you throw into your vision of yourself as a success, the more vibrant and alive the image will become in your mind, and the easier it will be to work toward making it a reality.
- **Don't just see it—feel it.** You need to associate emotions with the things you're imagining for yourself. By attaching your honest, innermost feelings to your vision, it will become more real to you.
- **Sense it.** Engage your physiology. I want you to feel the physi-

cal sensations in the vision. Feel the road pounding under your feet as you cross the line at the marathon. Feel the power in your shoulders as you hoist your toddler onto your shoulders after a round of tag at the playground. Attaching physical actions to your mental musings will help make them all the more familiar and real and will help you focus your everyday actions.

- **Put it on paper.** This one has been around for a while, but it's worth doing and putting some energy into it. Why? Because it works! Take the vision you've created in your head and give it life; some people call this a "vision board." Make a collage of the things you want the most. It can exist on a posterboard in your office or as the screensaver on your computer. It's a fun exercise. Bottom line: the greater your exposure to your wants and desires, the better chance you'll give yourself of attaining them.

FLIP THE SCRIPT •• 2 POINTS

Words are powerful. The things you say are what you believe. What you believe, you do. And what you do creates your reality. For this reason, the language you use must be geared toward positivity and success, not negativity and failure. Remove words like *can't* from your vocabulary. And pay close attention to your choice of adjectives. Instead of saying something's *hard,* say it's *not easy.* Instead of saying something's *impossible,* say it's a *challenge.* Don't say you're *trying* (the word *try* means you're planning on failing); instead say you're *doing.* Don't say you're *bad at* something; say you're *working on* it or *learning* it. Trust me, these small shifts make a huge difference in the way you perceive the world.

DON'T BE A PERFECTIONIST ••• 3 POINTS

Why should you not strive to be perfect? Because no one is! You'll surely set yourself up to fail, if you believe that you can or must be perfect all the time. Jettison that all-or-nothing mentality. If you fall off the wagon, which at one point or another you will, just let it go. Steer yourself in the right direction, and move on.

It's always amazed me how people can eat well and work out religiously for weeks at a time, then one day when they're stressed, they'll have some pizza or other junk they've been craving. Their entire regimen—eating, exercising, attitude—goes to hell. The little blip gets blown out of all proportion and triggers a wave of self-loathing and bingeing. Have some perspective, please!

Here's an analogy that I use a lot, and I want you to remember it for when this scenario happens to you. If you get a flat tire, you don't get out of the car and flatten all three of the other tires, do you? Hell no! You get out, change the flat, and keep going. The same rule applies to your lifestyle. Pick yourself up, dust yourself off, get back on the wagon, and keep moving forward. Keep perspective in your pocket, and leave perfectionism alone.

STRIP • 1 POINT

If you're having a hard time getting motivated, strip down to your undies and face yourself in the mirror. I'm not asking you to pick yourself apart and criticize every real or imagined flaw. Instead, I want you to look at where you are currently, level with yourself, and say, "No, I really don't want to paint that doughnut to the back of my ass. And yes, I could probably use a workout right now." Accept your state of affairs, get out of denial, take responsibility, and choose to make a change. Acceptance is extremely liberating; it can help you let go of many of the insecurities that will hold you back, if you let them. You can't look at yourself clearly if you're hiding behind your clothing.

Now I want you to dump all the frumpy clothes that allow you to conceal your body. Get rid of them once and for all, so you can't hide behind them anymore.

LIVE VICARIOUSLY • 1 POINT

Read about, watch, or listen to someone else's slim success story; it'll be inspirational. Look at before-and-after pictures on the web (I have a ton of these testimonials for Body Revolution on www .jillianmichaels.com) or watch *The Biggest Loser*. It doesn't really matter whose story it is, where you find it, or how you digest it. All that matters is that you learn about and experience another person's journey—follow his or her struggles and ultimate success. We humans are good at identifying with others. When we see someone else achieve their goal, it helps to motivate us. It cultivates our ability to believe in ourselves, to realize that we too can achieve a lofty goal.

CREATE A MANTRA • 1 POINT

I think most mantras are sappy platitudes that barely scratch the surface of self-worth, but there's a way to make them a valuable, powerful, and positive tool. The key is to make your mantra a short, simple, action-oriented statement that becomes a rule you live by. Although it's hard to create deep meaning in one sentence, it's possible. Don't pick a mantra that you think you *should* be saying to yourself, like "Just love yourself" or "Smile" or "See the glass as half full." These are stupid choices—you should already know them, and so you won't need them as a mantra. Instead, pick something you've heard that drives you and connects with you deeply. Pick a rule you can live by that makes you and your life better.

Lately, my mantra has been "A goal without a plan is just a dream." I remind myself of this whenever I get impulsive or impatient. It slows me down and reminds me that some of the things we most desire in life take time to come to fruition. The rule grounds me and keeps me proactive and focused.

You don't have to force yourself to come up with something spectacular. When you hear a phrase or a saying that resonates with you, make it your mantra. Repeat it to yourself when you're in doubt, or when you need a little reminder of how or why to do something important to you (like living slim). It will help keep you inspired.

SET THE STAGE • • • 3 POINTS

Have you ever heard the cliché "You're a product of your environment"? Well, it's true of all of us, to a certain extent. Our environments can strongly influence our thoughts, choices, and performance in life. Since our entire modern culture is set up as an "environmental obesogen," setting up your own personal environment for success, not sabotage, is crucial.

Look around you, at your work space, living space, car, and any other location where you spend time. Take note of anything and everything that might undermine your slim lifestyle. It could be the Dunkin' Donuts on your route to work that always manages to lure you. Maybe it's the bagels in your office kitchen or the candy bowl on your coworker's desk. Wherever you identify these saboteurs, do your best to remove, replace, or circumvent them. Take an alternate route to work, one that steers clear of the doughnut shop. Bring your own food, and avoid the office kitchen like the plague. Converse via e-mail or phone with the coworker who is stocking fattening snacks; stay out of his or her office. Once you change your habits, and your environment, it's a good chance they'll stay changed. Habit is that powerful.

Surround yourself with inspirational images (like the vision board we discussed earlier or your goal-weight-loss outfit). Watch TV shows that lift your spirits. Read books and magazines that are positive, with strong messages of hope and self-empowerment, like *A New Earth, Men's Health, The Four Agreements, O,* or *Shape.* Leave your running shoes by the door in the morning so you're incentivized to grab a workout on your lunch hour. Using your physical space to automate healthy behaviors is one of the easiest and most profound changes you can make in your life. So get on it!

BUILDING SUPPORT

MAKE AN ANNOUNCEMENT • • • 3 POINTS

In a recent survey by Medi-Weightloss Clinics, 53 percent of women said that others had pressured them to eat foods that weren't on their diet. Fifty-six percent of those women said they caved because they didn't want to insult the person offering food. Forty-one percent said they caved because they didn't want to call attention to their diet. Thirty-five percent said it was because others made jokes about their diet. What am I going to say? *These are just excuses for not taking control of your life and health.* Unacceptable excuses. Grow a frigging backbone! Speak up for yourself! Who else will, if you won't? Be direct, and let others know about your slim goal. That will help hold you accountable with all your friends (those who are supportive and those who aren't), allowing you to recruit the encouragement you need from those closest to you. And it will force those who sabotage you to face up to their own behavior and hopefully shame them into stopping.

COMMUNICATE YOUR NEEDS • • • 3 POINTS

People aren't mind readers. Oftentimes friends or family can sabotage your slim without consciously realizing it. Don't assume they know what you need or how to give it to you—you'll just end up disappointed when you don't get it. Whether it's the coworkers who keep dragging you out for drinks after work, or the boyfriend who orders pizza in every night, or the mom who keeps baking you cookies—tell them about your goal. Start by telling them how important being healthy and slim is to you. Then tell them *how* they can help you. I want you to literally give them the tools and communicate to them the exact ways you need them to encourage and support you.

Tell your mom to come up with skinny treat recipes instead of fattening ones. Tell your boyfriend you want him to work out with you and go out for sushi afterward. Tell the coworkers that you're not boozing right now, but you'd love to catch a movie or hit the gym with them. You *can* bring them around to a place of support instead of sabotage. Once you empower the people closest to you with strategies and knowledge of your needs, you'll be amazed at what a huge difference it makes in your ability to stick with it and go after your goals in a huge way.

SUPPORT GOES TWO WAYS • • • 3 POINTS

This is a big one. One of the main reasons people cite for abandoning their slimming efforts is that their significant other wasn't on the same page about lifestyle, goals, and values. I've found that this dilemma often extends beyond romantic relationships, crossing over into relationships with parents and close friends. This problem is almost identical to the one we covered in "Communicate your needs," but it's about what you do when that advice doesn't work. When it doesn't, there's usually a big reason why—perhaps the other party feels threatened on some level that if you get healthy, you'll outgrow them, not need them, or perhaps they fear that your newfound healthiness will incite questions about their own lack of healthy habits. While such fears may not be rational, they're still real.

The best thing you can do is open up a dialogue with the person(s) again, reiterating what you want and why you want it. Then be sure to tell them how much you love them and how important they are to you. Over time, as they begin to feel safe and secure with "the new you," I predict they'll eventually come around, and maybe even jump on your healthy bandwagon.

CLEAN HOUSE—HATERS HAVE TO GO • • • 3 POINTS

The number-one tenet when building a support system is this: everyone you invite into your life should make you better. When handpicking your entourage, the people with whom you spend the bulk of your time, you must follow this rule. Hang out only with people for whom your success is their success. The people around you should support your quest to be great—or they should be gone! It's time to reevaluate your life and take inventory of who is on your team and who isn't. Clear all nonsupportive, toxic people out of your life. All the jealous friends who sabotage you must go. Ultimately, we are the company we keep. That means haters and enablers—you're out of here.

SET BOUNDARIES • • • 3 POINTS

Consider this the fourth step in a series of self-support must-do's. The series starts with (1) communicating your needs, (2) validating and supporting your loved ones, and (3) cleaning house if the first two steps fail.

But if the toxic person is one who can't be removed (like a family member), we must resort to setting firm, ironclad boundaries. If you and your mother fight because she thinks your healthy diet is "silly," then don't eat with her. If your sister makes fun of you hitting the gym while you're home for the holidays, don't tell her where you're going. Look for the "hot spots" in the relationship, and avoid them. Some subjects will instigate fighting and sabotage and leave you feeling crappy. Sidestep them at all costs. Instead, steer the relationship and your communications toward positive and neutral topics, ones that don't incite quarrels and insecurities, yours or theirs.

You can and should be direct with your family members, by the way, about your needs and limits. Let them know that you don't want to discuss the topic with them. If they don't hear you or respect your boundaries and start in on you anyway, tell them you love them, but you're going to leave or hang up until they choose to have respectful regard for your position. You're not abandoning them; you're simply maximizing the positive in the relationship and minimizing the negative. I guarantee that after you continue this healthy pattern of interacting several times, they'll get the message, and you'll have bought yourself some breathing room.

GET YOUR BACK • • • 3 POINTS

Be your own best friend. *How do I become a better friend to myself?* you ask. You do it by learning to put yourself in the best position to succeed. Great leaders work to create an environment that is conducive to their employees' success. Similarly, being your own best friend means setting yourself up for success as you accept the challenge for greatness (and slimness). It's all about self-acceptance. If you feel worthy of what you're aspiring to and pay yourself the same respect and love you would to others, you'll get where you need to go.

Here's what I mean. Years ago I was in therapy bitching about how I did everything for everyone else and no one did anything for me. While I was mid–pity party, my shrink interrupted me. He told me that it wasn't everyone else who was letting me down; I was doing it. I protested and called him crazy, but he went on to prove his point. He listed all the loving things I did for others and showed how I never did those same things for myself. The implication clearly was that when I started giving myself all the things I gave to others, my life would be immeasurably richer. The attention and help I got from the outside world would be a bonus.

I took his advice. I bought flowers for my bedroom. I got myself a massage. I rented the movie that I wanted to watch. I took care of myself. I made time for myself. I referred to myself in respectful, loving ways. And you know what? My life changed in amazing ways—forever. After I began to do that, not by coincidence, I started attracting more supportive, loving people into my life. I was happier. I felt stronger. I had more confidence and subsequently more strength to take risks and "shoot for the stars." While I know this may sound somewhat silly and reminiscent of a bad *Saturday Night Live* skit, it works.

Look at all the things you do for your parents, kids, significant other, or best friend. I bet you even help out your neighbors and coworkers more often than you help yourself. Now I want you to make a conscious effort to treat yourself in the exact same loving and giving ways. Then watch how your attitude, motivation, and slim status all change for the better.

ACCENTUATE THE NEGATIVE •• 2 POINTS

My sage advice is to ignore the haters. Suze Orman once said to me, "The elephants keep walking, while the dogs keep barking." She meant, don't let small-minded, jealous people stop you from achieving your goals.

Maybe you've heard another saying: "Success is the greatest revenge"? Some people get motivated by naysayers—they get jazzed to prove that those who say "No, you can't!" are dead wrong. Have you ever heard Lady Gaga or Katy Perry talk about how so many told each of them they wouldn't make it? These two superstars are now on top of the world in their careers and fame, with more money than they probably know what to do with each day. They can turn up their noses at those who didn't believe in them.

My business partner is a person who doesn't accept the negative or ever feel defeated. He loves it when people say no to him or to our company because he relishes the opportunity to prove them wrong. If you can't let go of someone's negativity or nastiness toward you, then channel it. Instead of letting it get you down, let it drive you forward and propel you to success.

ASK FOR FEEDBACK •• 2 POINTS

One of the best tools to employ when you're attempting to learn, grow, or improve in any area of your life is to have a coach or mentor as part of your go-to team. This is someone who not only supports you but has the information you need in order to succeed; someone who can show you where you're going wrong and how to turn it around so you can ultimately get it right. I've been this person for many people, and I can right years of wrongdoing in a matter of seconds because of my expertise in health and wellness.

Don't suffer unnecessarily. If you can't lock a friend in to help you on a permanent basis, hire a trainer or a registered dietitian for a session or two. Let a professional analyze and assess what you've been doing; they can help you make a few tweaks that will give you a jump-start if you need one. While I'm hoping this book will give you all you need, a little one-on-one personalized advice for a specific or unique issue can sometimes go a long way.

BLOG • 1 POINT

Write a blog about your experiences. Read blogs that inspire you. As I said earlier, reading others' success stories is motivating. Sharing your story with others can be a giveback—as well as a way to garner support from others who are experiencing similar hardships or challenges.

BE A TEAM PLAYER • 1 POINT

It's amazing how much help message boards and online communities can provide when you're living slim. Some people I've worked with who long ago hit their weight-loss goals still subscribe to my website www.jillianmichaels.com—they remain members simply to be active and connected with others on my message boards. A Web environment provides you with anonymity. You can speak freely without worrying about who will know or judge you, and it offers support from people who

---

SLIM MYTH:

High-fructose corn syrup is no worse for you than table sugar.

FAST FACT: NOT TRUE! The people who make high-fructose corn syrup (HFCS) have tried to spin it and say it's the same as sugar. While chemically similar, our bodies don't process them in the same way. HFCS is processed only by the liver, whereas sugar is metabolized by every cell in the body. That's why HFCS is a greater contributor to obesity, high triglycerides, diabetes, fatty liver disease, and the like. Don't get me wrong—I'm not giving you free license to binge on sugar. You should still use it only in moderation. But avoid HFCS at all costs.

are going through similar things. It's a buddy system that also helps to hold you accountable. There are many different options out there. My suggestion is surf the Web. Look for the environment where you feel the most comfortable, and start making friends!

EAT RIGHT, MOVE MORE

LISTEN UP • • • 3 POINTS

Nothing scares me straight like a conversation with my doctor. When I learned from my doc that I was an estrogen-dominant female who was at high risk for breast cancer and that alcohol significantly increased that risk, I practically went cold turkey.

When it comes to slim, it's actually not just about skinny jeans, bikinis, and sex with the lights on. Slim goes way deeper and is directly associated with the quality of your health and subsequently the quality of your life. Go see your doctor, and get your numbers checked: cholesterol, blood sugar, blood pressure, resting heart rate. Then allow your physician to give you the lecture about how dangerous the bad numbers are and how much better every aspect of your wellness will be when you drop, or keep off, the excess pounds for good.

MAKE IT TASTY • 1 POINT

You'd probably be a lot more motivated to eat healthy and slimming foods if they tasted good, right? Well, there's no rule in the universe that says they can't. There are plenty of tasty and healthy treats that help to build a healthy body and mind. (Refer back to the "Get Cooking" tips in Chapter 3.) I want you to be creative with your recipes. I've had roasted brussels sprouts that were just as tasty as mashed potatoes. It's all in the prep. So do your homework and experiment with healthy foods until you establish some tasty slimming dishes that you enjoy and look forward to eating. Here's a sample treat done slim to get you started:

ICE CREAM SLIMWICH (120 CALORIES PER 'WICH)

¾ cup ricotta cheese

1½ tablespoons mashed raspberries (or other mashable fruit of your choice)

1 tablespoon raw brown sugar

1 tablespoon dark chocolate chips

16 chocolate graham crackers

In a small bowl, stir together ricotta, mashed fruit, and sugar. When fully blended, fold in the chocolate chips. Place 8 crackers on a rimmed baking sheet. Divide the mixture evenly onto the crackers. Top with the remaining crackers and freeze for at least an hour. Once frozen, wrap each Slimwich separately in protective wrap; they'll keep for up to a week in the freezer.

INUNDATE YOURSELF •• 2 POINTS

Surround yourself with images that inspire you to get slim. Post them on your fridge, desktop, and car dashboard. Place them on any surface you might see before you make a food choice. When I was a kid trying to get in shape, I put up a picture of Linda Hamilton from *Terminator 2.* (Remember what sick shape she was in? Her arms are legendary to this day!) Every time I wanted to reach for a piece of pizza or a doughnut, I looked at that picture, and it inspired me to change my mind. I look at pictures of Madonna now, hot in her fifties with a body to die for, and I put down the extra cookie or glass of wine instantly. While I don't want you to get in the habit of looking outside yourself for motivation, there's something to be said for stories and images that can catalyze us to take action. Pick out individuals or imagery that helps you achieve your slim agenda and surround yourself with them.

DRESS FOR SUCCESS •• 2 POINTS

Buy a goal outfit that flatters your physique. We used to do this on *Biggest Loser* back in the early seasons, and I can't for the life of me figure out or remember why we stopped. We would have the contestants pick an outfit they wanted to fit into, and we'd display it for them in a case. I'm not saying you need to build a shrine to the outfit in your bedroom, but maybe hang it in on the back of your door so you can see it. When you're contemplating whether to get your sweat on, take a look at that outfit and picture yourself in it. I'm willing to bet it gives you the little push you need to move your butt!

BE A KID AGAIN •• 2 POINTS

Whenever the thought of doing a structured workout seems like torture to me, I find ways of being active that are fun. One of my tricks is to act like a kid again. I take a snowboarding lesson, or a surfing lesson, or I go paddleboarding. Try it. Skateboard to your office, or bike to run your errands. Go bowling with friends. You get the idea. Ultimately, having fun like this will be great for your spirit and your body.

KEEP IT SOCIAL •• 2 POINTS

Working out can sometimes feel tedious, but it can be more palatable when you make it social. As they say, misery loves company. Kidding—sorta. A partner inspires progress. And if you really hate exercise, commiserating *is* much better than going solo.

Here are some ideas for keeping it social:

- **Get a buddy.** Your buddy could be a coworker or another mom at your kid's school. Maybe it's a neighbor, a family member, or a lifelong friend. Simply let them know you're going on a health kick, and see who wants to kick it with you.

- **Join a running or biking group.** This is a great way to make new friends, learn a new sport, and get and stay in slim mode.
- **Look for organized fitness activities** in your city or neighborhood, such as basketball or softball games. Search the Internet to see what's available. You'll be surprised how popular such sports are for grown-ups, and by how easy it is to find a team. If nothing online or locally offered appeals to you, start your own group or team.
- **Take a class.** Fitness classes can become a culture and community unto themselves, like the CrossFit Junkies and the Zumba Addicts. Even if you're not looking to join a cult, a class is a great way to compete with others, stay motivated, and socialize.

GEEK OUT •• 2 POINTS

Treat yourself to a cool fitness gadget like a heart rate monitor, pedometer, or waterproof headphones. There are gadgets galore to give you feedback, motivate you, train you, and make your workout more efficient or pleasurable. Many gadgets provide you with personal info, which can be very incentivizing. The BodyMedia Armband will show you how many calories you're burning from minute to minute throughout the day; it's only natural to set goals with it. If you burned 1,800 yesterday, you'll probably want to shoot for 2,000 tomorrow, and so on.

You can also download fitness apps from iTunes. My Slim-Down Solution app will gives you workouts, recipes, a calorie counter, and more. I love the app Strava for cycling, and also Running Coach's Clipboard. The possibilities for apps are endless. They have ones for yoga, Pilates, dance, gymnastics, and rowing—anything and everything you can think of.

Apps and gadgets give you something new to play with, and because you're excited to use them, you keep up with your workouts. My Strava app, for example, shows me how far I biked, how many feet I climbed, and how long it took me. So the next time I go for a ride, I'm out to beat my best time.

JAM OUT •• 2 POINTS

Get your workout playlist together. I'm serious. Studies have shown that people who exercise to music they love will work harder and for a longer time—they'll put in up to 10 percent more effort and gain 15 percent more endurance. One study interviewed 2,000 individuals across the United States and found that 94 percent of those who exercised with music said they would never exercise without it. The same study found that music users feel they're more likely to exercise when they're *not* in the mood if they know the music is available. Apparently, the sound of the music blocks our nerves from signaling body fatigue and decreases our perception of our exercise effort.

Another study, geared toward measuring weight loss in women, determined that those who walked to music lost significantly more weight and body fat. Additionally, the music-listening group adhered better to the program, and fewer of them dropped out of the study. I know personally that a good tune will always inspire me to run faster and longer. While you can, of course, listen to whatever music *you* love that gets you going, there's a suggested ideal rhythm of music for fitness, which is 140 to 160 beats per minute (BPM). If you don't know what 160 beats per minute sounds like, check out Runningplaylist.net. It has more than 100 playlists, ranging from alternative to pop, and it cites the BPM for each song. In addition, I

SLIM MYTH:
Certain types of training can lengthen your muscles.
FAST FACT: It's physically impossible to lengthen a muscle after you're fully grown. Muscles have a fixed origin and insertion point, so although you may feel longer and leaner after a yoga class or a Pilates workout, probably the fact that you're leaner, more flexible, and more fit is giving you the illusion of having longer muscles.

create a new workout list monthly on my site, and my business partner, Giancarlo, who doubles as a DJ, creates a free downloadable exercise mix for my Facebook fans every month. Be sure to check it out and pack your iPod with these song recommendations.

BE TRENDY • 1 POINT

Try a fad workout like pole fitness, a barre class, punk rope, ballroom dancing, or drum training to keep your fitness routines fresh. This will not only keep your training well rounded, it will fend off boredom, train the same muscles in a different way for a totally new experience, and help you find new things you're passionate about. It's sort of like a mini-adventure every time you train.

BE A FRONT-RUNNER •• 2 POINTS

Don't hide out in the back of your fitness class. Sit in the front row of your yoga, Pilates, or studio cycling class. The heat is on because you'll have to set the example for the people behind you, and you'll do no screwing around as you're directly in the teacher's line of sight. Being up front gives you the inspiration to go for it, and the oomph to keep going when you want to quit.

SHOOT IT • 1 POINT

Take before, during (monthly), and after pics or video log your efforts and success. This is a big one. If you've followed my programs before, you know I've insisted upon it both in my Body Revolution ninety-day weight-loss DVD program and in my book *Making the Cut*. Here's why: the before picture will show you how far you've come. It's easy, along the way, to lose track of how much success you've already achieved. When you have a week where the scale doesn't move, or you just need a frame of reference, the before pic will remind you of your accomplishments to date and boost your spirits. It's a great way to measure your progress and will remind you why you started your new lifestyle in the first place.

START A REWARDS PROGRAM • • • 3 POINTS

Plan on doing something special when you achieve your goal, so you'll have something to look forward to that will drive you to cross the finish line. It could be big like a beach vacation or small like a pedicure. Try to make the reward correspond to the accomplishment of a wellness goal. For example, decide that if you hit the gym four times this week, you'll give yourself a mani/pedi on Saturday. If you lose the last 20 pounds, you'll take that beach holiday you've been dreaming about forever. Having additional positive incentives can go a long way when it comes to staying motivated.

GIVE BACK • 1 POINT

Many of my friends have signed up for charity rides or runs. I did the Stand Up to Cancer Malibu Triathlon. Another friend of mine did the AIDS Ride. Yet another did a 100-mile bike ride to raise money to fight cancer for Livestrong. The key here is that signing up both obligates and motivates you, since you're doing it for a cause.

OFF TO THE RACES • 1 POINT

One of the hottest trends in fitness these days is the fitness event where individuals can test their athleticism and physical toughness. Maybe you've heard of the Warrior Dash (www.warriordash .com), the Spartan Race (www.spartanrace.com), or Tough Mudder (www.toughmudder.com), to name a few. Maybe you'll want to try one. The idea is to incentivize yourself with a goal that drives you to be the best you can be—to push yourself and defy your limits. These races are *not* for everyone, but for those of you who are goal-oriented and love a challenge: pick a race and start training for it. Make sure, though, that you select a competition where you can give yourself enough lead time to properly train and be prepped and ready to compete.

DEDICATE THE DEED • 1 POINT

This one works really well on my *Biggest Loser* contestants. I help them create mental motivators by dedicating milestones of their workout to someone or something important to them. Try it out. Dedicate a mile out of your jog to your son, or do a circuit from your workout in honor of your significant other. You get the idea. Although you and your best life should always be your greatest motivator, it's important to remember that the slimmer and health-ier you are, the better mom, husband, parent, friend, child, worker, and all-around person you'll be to the important people in your life.

LET LOVE MOVE YOU • • 2 POINTS

Collect inspirational notes from people you love and post them on your treadmill. Or take a picture of your loved one and look at it on your phone during your workout. I do this with my kids all the time. I snap their pic, then use my iPhone for listening to tunes when I train. Right there are their little faces, reminding me that I need to be around for them for years and years to come.

TAKE BABY STEPS • • 2 POINTS

Do you remember that movie *What About Bob*? (If you're too young to get this reference—damn you, youngster!) On the days when you just can't imagine getting to the gym, do a little negotiation with yourself. Give yourself permission to do just 1 mile on the treadmill, or just a 20-minute circuit block on the gym floor. Then get up and go. Once you get there and get the blood pumping and the feel-good brain chemicals flowing, you'll likely be inclined to dig in and knock out an additional 15 minutes before you finish your workout. I've seen it happen over and over. Give yourself permission to do less, and more often than not you'll end up doing as much, if not more, than you expected.

ADD IT UP, DROP IT OFF

GIVE YOURSELF 3 POINTS

- Make it personal.
- Establish your agenda.
- Behold the power of the pyramid.
- Paint a picture.
- Don't be a perfectionist.
- Set the stage.
- Make an announcement.
- Communicate your needs.
- Support goes two ways.
- Clean house—haters have to go.
- Set boundaries.
- Get your back.
- Listen up.
- Start a rewards program.

GIVE YOURSELF 2 POINTS

- Flip the script.
- Accentuate the negative.
- Ask for feedback.
- Inundate yourself.
- Dress for success.
- Be a kid again.
- Keep it social.
- Geek out.
- Jam out.

- Be a front-runner.
- Let love move you.
- Take baby steps.

GIVE YOURSELF 1 POINT

- Strip.
- Live vicariously.
- Create a mantra.
- Blog.
- Be a team player.
- Make it tasty.
- Be trendy.
- Shoot it.
- Give back.
- Off to the races.
- Dedicate the deed.

_____ **Total *points* for Chapter 5**

_____ **Total number of *tips* I'm incorporating**

CHAPTER 6

EVADING PITFALLS

Do you ever feel like the odds are stacked against you? Well, not to make you feel paranoid or anything, but sometimes when it comes to weight loss and health, they are. Between accessibility, time management, funds, and conflicting agendas, it can be pretty tough to lose weight. You can bypass these troublesome traps and get the results you're looking for with the right tools and strategies.

Let me say before we get down to business that it's okay to struggle. So often we feel shame when we struggle, as though it makes us less in some way. Many people have irrational thoughts like *If I were stronger, this wouldn't be a problem for me* or *If I were more disciplined, I wouldn't get strung up by that.* Utter crap. Struggle is part of life. The key is what you do with your struggles. And don't get it twisted—being strong and disciplined is great, but if you don't have the proper knowledge and information, you're screwed anyway. So in this chapter I'm going to make sure you have all the info you need to combat these demons in the most effective way possible.

Let's kick it off with the top slim traps: hunger and cravings. I'll arm you with any and every piece of advice or actionable step available to fend off these weight-loss demons (other than surgery and drugs—which are bad, by the way).

··

Handling Hunger

THINK IT THROUGH • • • 3 POINTS

There's an Alcoholics Anonymous tip that says "Think through the drink." That is, *before* you drink, think through how it will play out if you actually have even a sip. I've found this tip works exceptionally well with food binges, too. Before you indulge, think it all the way through. How will you feel five minutes after you've eaten the food? How about the next morning? Better yet, how about in a year, after you've thrown down lots of excess calories unnecessarily over the months and have packed on 10 extra pounds? This one gets me to put the fork down every time.

TAKE INVENTORY • • • 3 POINTS

Most people *think* they're physically hungry when they aren't. When you're not sure if something else is prodding you to eat, ask yourself the following questions:

1. When was the last time I ate?

2. Am I experiencing physical signs of hunger like light-headedness, mood swings, and tummy growling?

3. Am I having trouble thinking or making a decision? Am I cranky?

If you've eaten a substantial meal within the last 3 hours and you aren't actually having any physical symptoms of hunger, then chances are . . . you're not hungry! Ask yourself what else could be going on; what emotion is masquerading as hunger? Are you stressed, bored, lonely, or angry? Write down what you're feeling and why you're feeling it. Then try to resolve the actual issue in an appropriate way rather than relying on food as the solution.

CHECK FOR THIRST • • • 3 POINTS

It's not uncommon for dehydration to disguise itself as hunger. If you find yourself feeling hungry, drink a glass of water first to make sure you're not dehydrated. Wait 15 to 20 minutes—if you're still hungry, eat. As a rule of thumb, drink first, eat later; you'll avoid packing on unwanted pounds.

SHOUT IT FROM THE MOUNTAINTOPS • • • 3 POINTS

If you're about to eat something you know you'll regret later, like a huge bag of chips, before you mindlessly down it, stop and say out loud: "I'm eating this entire bag of chips because I'm bored, sad, mad, [insert emotion here], and I'm not even hungry. I know I'm going to mentally beat myself up afterward. I'm consciously making the decision to worsen my health and take a sledgehammer to my weight-loss aspirations." If you do this, there's a good chance you'll think better of your decision. Sometimes when you bring things out into the open in this way, it takes you out of an unconscious, impulsive behavior that will mess you up and brings you to a supportive place of reason and logic.

....

SLIM MYTH:
Some foods have "negative calories."

FAST FACT: We've talked about free foods, and they're awesome choices for curbing hunger. But the theory we are dispelling here is that your body uses *more* calories to digest them than they contain, so you burn calories just from eating them. That's not true. These foods are extremely low calorie, and you can pretty much eat as much of them as you want and never gain a pound, but digesting them won't actually create a calorie deficit.

....

SLOW YOUR ROLL • • 2 POINTS

An *American Journal of Clinical Nutrition* study showed that when you chew your food slowly and completely, as opposed to scarfing it, you take in nearly 12 percent fewer calories. It takes the body 20 minutes to register feelings of fullness—you know this, but you may not have considered how advantageous it is to slow down. Eat slowly, and you'll give yourself a chance to feel full before you've scarfed an entire pizza. Try these simple strategies to go into slow mo and save yourself some calories and an expanding waistline:

- Eat with your opposite hand.
- Chew your food till it's the consistency of applesauce.
- Take a sip of water between bites.
- Consume slow foods, like pistachios or peel-and-eat shrimp.
- Cut your food into small bites.

Although some of these ideas may seem tedious or make you feel silly when doing them, that won't matter when you're rockin' that hot dress on a Friday night.

EAT FOR FREE • • • 3 POINTS

Did you ever play the game that asks, If you could have one wish, what would it be? My answer was always the ability to eat whatever I wanted and never gain weight. I've had no such luck with that so far, but there's such a thing as free food, at least where your waist-line is concerned. I'm talking about high-fiber, high-water-content, nutrient-dense, extremely low-calorie foods that take *nearly* as many calories for your body to digest as the amount of calories they actually contain. What I love about these foods is that you can fill up on them when you're hungry—I mean literally eat as much of them as you want (provided you don't add fattening sauces, oils, or dressings) and not gain weight.

I'm referring to these foods:

Bell peppers	Jicama
Broccoli	Kale
Brussels sprouts	Leafy greens
Cabbage	Lettuce
Cauliflower	Mushrooms
Celery	Snap peas
Cucumbers	Zucchini
Green beans	

I know. I built this one up as if I were going to tell you I'd discovered a calorie-free cake. Instead I hit you with rabbit food. This
advice, however, has gotten me through many hungry nights.
When my appetite is out of control and I'm out to dinner, I order

....

SLIM MYTH:
Exercise makes you eat more.

FAST FACT: Many studies have found just the opposite, that exercise *suppresses*
food intake. In 2012 researchers looked at how exercise affects our hunger hormones. It seems the relationship between appetite hormones, and the brain's
response to food sensory cues, is dependent on *the type* of exercise you do. Back
in 2008, a U.K. study found that cardio training is more effective than resistance
training in suppressing hunger for two hours after training, due to hormonal
changes in the release of ghrelin and peptide YY. Ghrelin, a hunger-stimulating
hormone, decreased in both activities, but only peptide YY, which suppresses
hunger, decreased during cardio. A recent 2012 study, published in the *Journal of
Applied Physiology*, found that exercise significantly lowers our response to food cues
after exercise. The evidence suggests that exercise may lessen your desire to eat by
altering how certain parts of your brain, what is aptly called the food-reward network, respond to the sight of food. Bottom line: Don't be afraid to work out! It helps
you eat less and burns extra calories.

....

three veggie sides, like steamed spinach with lemon, steamed brussels sprouts (that I dip in hot sauce), steamed green beans, and for my meal an enormous dinner salad. Then I power through all and eat only a bite of dessert. It fills me up without the calories and squashes my hunger.

REMEMBER THE RULES • • • 3 POINTS

Sorry for being redundant, but I cannot tell you this rule often enough because breaking it can lead to a pitfall tumble. DO NOT SKIP MEALS, especially breakfast! I mentioned this in the four-by-four rule in Chapter 1. When you skip meals, you crash your blood sugar, which inhibits willpower, and from a physiological perspective it actually makes food taste better to you. This, of course, causes you to eat too much of the wrong things. Don't be an idiot. Don't skip meals.

BUST A MOOD • 1 POINT

Researchers suggest that when you're happier and more content, you have less of a tendency to overeat. One study on how mood affects food choice found that feeling angry can increase comfort- and impulsive-eating behaviors. Another study observed individuals' emotional response while watching a happy or sad movie; it found that the subjects watching the sad movie wanted to eat comfort (aka unhealthy) food like buttered popcorn and consumed more of it than those viewing the upbeat movie, who ate less food and made healthier food choices. A 2010 study, conducted at the University of Southampton in the U.K., found that a negative mood increased people's desire for food, as well as the urge to reward themselves through eating. I'm sure you've lived what the researchers documented—who hasn't?

Being chipper all the time is easier said than done, I know. We all have those days, but making an effort to make yourself happy, smile more, and do more of the things you love can actually help you curb your appetite. Keeping a more positive attitude will not only help you lose weight, it will also help you keep the weight off. On even your worst day, I bet if you tried, you could find something good that has happened. Before you reach for food, focus on all the things that went well that day. They don't have to be big to make you feel better.

POUND THE PAVEMENT •• 2 POINTS

Research published in the journal *Appetite* suggests that a 15-minute walk can keep your mind off snacking. The next time you're thinking of having that pint of ice cream, before you scarf down a ton of calories that you'll be sorry for, hit the road. Walk the dog for 15 minutes. Take a stroll around the neighborhood with your kid. If you live in a walking city like New York, run an errand on foot. I don't care how you do it—just do it. It took me a while to personally buy into this one, even with the research, but then I tried it and found that the majority of the time, I had a positive result. If you want to quell hunger—get movin'! Just don't walk to a fast-food joint or mini-market!

BE A LITTLE NUTTY • 1 POINT

Eat 5 walnuts or 8 almonds before a meal (roughly 65 calories) to stimulate production of cholecystokinin, a hormone that slows your stomach from emptying. This trick allows you to stay fuller longer from your meals. Remember, though, that each walnut has about 15 calories and each almond has 8, so incorporate the additions into your daily calorie allowance.

KEEP IT COOL • 1 POINT

Studies show that cool colors suppress appetite while warm colors increase it. That's why all those fast-food joints are themed in yellow, orange, and red. Hello Golden Arches. So while Big Food is using this information to wreck your diet and grab your cash, you can use it proactively to achieve the opposite goal. Use blue plates. Drink from purple cups. Paint your kitchen green—well, maybe you don't have to paint the walls green (that could be a little overwhelming). Try just laying out some green placemats the next time you eat, paired with your blue plates and utensils. That's more easily managed.

OUT OF SIGHT—OUT OF MIND • • • 3 POINTS

Remove food from your sight. It's less about hunger than about willpower. We tend to eat things that are in front of us. It's amazing how many times I've said I wasn't hungry, but then a friend started to eat, and suddenly "I could eat, too." An even clearer example: Bob and I regularly keep a bag of Newman's Own peanut butter cookies in our makeup room. When it's out on the counter, we devour it by the end of the week. When it's tucked away in the cabinet, however, a month could go by, and we wouldn't have even opened that package.

Remember: out of sight—out of mind—out of mouth.

HAVE AN EMERGENCY PLAN • • • 3 POINTS

I don't know what part of the world you live in, but here in California we all have our "earthquake emergency plan." We know what we are going to do when the big one hits, where we are going to go, and how much water, cash, and canned food we will carry. Just as you would prepare for this type of emergency, I want you to ferret out the dangers in your slim regimen and preemptively batten down the diet hatches, so to speak.

Here are the steps I want you to take:

1. Look at your life and identify the ways you get into trouble and sabotage your slim.

2. Write all these issues down.

3. For each one, develop a plan, so when it arises, you have a go-to behavior to turn to instead of food.

For example, if you always eat when you're stressed, list ways you can nurture yourself that aren't food related (take a bubble bath, buy some new songs for your workout playlist from iTunes, or turn to a hobby you love). If you know that going home for the holidays to your family will make you feel bad and turn to food, then have a good buddy on call to help talk you off the ledge. If you eat when you're lonely, make plans to go out with friends as often as possible, so you avoid sitting home alone with your fridge

---

SLIM MYTH:
The more you sweat, the more calories you burn.

FAST FACT: Sweating is your body's way of cooling itself—that's all. True, you burn more calories when you work harder; your muscles put in more effort, and your heart beats faster. So sweating more might make you think you're working harder, but that's not always the case. In some instances, the exact opposite is true. Let's take hot yoga, for example. According to Bikram's Yoga College, a Bikram yoga class should be practiced in a room heated to around 105 degrees. That's plenty hot, but many teachers are known to crank the temperature up to as high as 115 degrees. While hot yoga has been trending for a while now and Bikram aficionados swear by its benefits, working in this kind of extreme heat can make you weak, dehydrated, dizzy, and fatigued—and boy, are you sweating. Conversely, when you do yoga in a room that's a more regulated, moderate temperature, you're able to work at a much higher intensity. Even though you aren't sweating as much, you're still burning far more calories than you do in the Bikram class. The same can be said of working out in sauna suits or exercising outside in hot weather. To get a real burn, put yourself in as comfortable an environment as possible, so that you can train at the highest intensity possible.

as your friend. You've heard it: failing to plan is planning to fail. So get strategizing.

TIVO IT • 1 POINT

Fast-forward through food commercials. (The Papa John's pizza one gets me every damn time.) Your best defense is to not watch them, or better yet, use the commercials for an exercise break. Nowadays you get about 4 minutes of commercials every time your favorite show breaks. Crunch until the end of the first commercial, do lunges during the second, crank out some jumping jacks through the third one, and do push-ups for the last. Do the math—by the time you've watched an hourlong show, you've exercised a good 20 minutes or so—a pretty good calorie exchange from just being a couch potato.

HEAT IT UP • 1 POINT

Spicy foods can reduce your appetite by increasing your body's nor-epinephrine and epinephrine levels. Canadian researchers found that people who ate appetizers with hot sauce ate *200 fewer calo-ries* than people who didn't use it. And another study in the *British Journal of Nutrition* found that women who added 2 teaspoons of dried red pepper flakes to their food ate fewer calories during the day. When you order ethnic, like Indian or Chinese, tell them you want it spicy, and be sure to add a little fire to your everyday dishes for the same benefit.

PRACTICE YOGA • 1 POINT

Yoga for weight loss—yes, it's true. Practicing yoga regularly may help suppress appetite and therefore promote weight loss. Accord-ing to research published in the *Journal of the American Dietetic Association*, those who regularly engaged in yoga seemed to be more aware of their eating habits. They were less likely to binge or eat mindlessly. The scientists did not find a similar association with other types of physical activity, such as walking or running. These findings suggest that learning to be more self-observant through yoga will spill over into being more aware of your eating habits, leading to healthier choices and weight loss, independent of yoga as a physical practice. If you're looking for a way to control mindless eating, add a yoga session or two to your weekly workouts.

SLIM MYTH:
Exercise can erase my bad
eating habits.
FAST FACT: You can eat your way through any amount of exercise. Think about it. Spend an hour on the treadmill, and you can burn 500 calories—basically that's a slice and a half of pizza, without any sides. You have to eat right *and* work out if you are going to see results. If you're doing one but not the other, chances are you won't gain weight but you probably won't lose either. To ensure success, cover all bases with a clean diet and a solid exercise regimen.

START WITH SOUP •• 2 POINTS
Stave off hunger by starting your meal with a cup of soup, broth, or broth with veggies. This can curb the tendency to overeat. Wait 10 to 15 minutes before you eat your main meal, and there's a good chance you'll eat a lot less. If you're making your own veggie-based, potassium-rich, low-sodium broth, use organic vegetables such as asparagus, zucchini, green beans, and celery—especially the leafy heart. Use greens of any kind, parsley especially, as they're naturally diuretic. Don't add salt. Do add natural seasonings such as black and cayenne pepper, turmeric, dried mustard, and lemon juice, and you're off to a filling, slimming start to any meal.

Crushing Cravings

Don't confuse hunger with cravings. They're very different. You can have cravings when you're not hungry—usually for something salty or sweet. If you treat cravings as if they're hunger, you'll eat and eat, hoping they'll abate—but to no avail. The following section is geared specifically at crushing cravings so they don't ruin all your hard work.

BYPASSING THE BINGE

PLAY A ZERO-SUM GAME • • • 3 POINTS

Think about the treat you're going to ingest, then figure out how many hours of exercise you will need to put in to counteract it. To help you figure this out, look up the food you're going to consume in your calorie-counting app or pocket calorie-counting book. Then imagine that you're exercising *intensely*, burning around 10 calories a minute (give or take). For example: if you had the Bloomin' Onion appetizer from Outback Steak House at around 1,800 calories, you'd need to run at a minimum of 7 mph for about 3 hours straight to work it off. That's practically a marathon. I play this game with myself all the time. You'll be amazed how quickly you write that junk food off. An hour and a half of intense circuit training for the Big Mac—I don't think so.

ENGAGE IN TEATIME • 1 POINT

This tip comes straight from the mouth of supermodel Naomi Campbell. She says that one of her top tricks for fending off hunger and cravings is to sip tea. There are a number of reasons why this works. First, many teas are lightly caffeinated; caffeine is a natural appetite suppressant. Green tea, for example, has been shown to squelch hunger, boost energy, burn up to 4 percent more calories, and increase the rate of fat oxidation (fat burning). Herbal teas (noncaffeinated) can also be helpful in fending off hunger, as some of the properties of herbals support a host of organ and metabolic functions.

Here are my top picks:

HERBAL OPTIONS

1. **Dandelion tea.** Dandelion is regaled for curbing cravings for sweets and is also reputed to boost metabolism, flush out the kidneys, and help treat digestive problems. You can purchase it at your local grocer or make it fresh from the dandelion root. It's most effective as a craving killer when consumed three times each day.

2. **Siberian ginseng.** Ginseng helps stabilize blood-sugar levels, which in turn helps stave off cravings and suppress appetite. People with a history of high blood pressure or anxiety must limit their consumption of Siberian ginseng, though, or find natural alternatives. This type of tea is commonly found in Asian grocers or herbal shops.

3. **Licorice tea.** This "sweet root" tea helps to sustain healthy blood sugar levels, reducing cravings for sweets and managing hunger.

4. **Bilberry tea.** Bilberry helps kill cravings, particularly in the evening, as it's both naturally decaffeinated and defends against sugar-induced munching. Bilberries have blood-sugar-balancing effects, like many of the other herbals listed here, which will send you running for that late-night snack far less often.

CAFFEINATED OPTIONS

1. **Green tea.** This wonder beverage helps boost metabolism and burn fat while simultaneously inhibiting hunger and cravings. It's also been shown to help lower cholesterol, prevent diabetes and stroke, and stave off dementia.

2. **Yerba maté.** This tea helps to suppress hunger, boost metabolism, and reduce fatigue.

3. **Black tea.** A study in the *Journal of American College of Nutrition* found that black tea decreases blood sugar levels by 10 percent for two and a half hours, so you'll feel fuller faster and avoid hunger later on.

PSYCH OUT YOUR TASTE BUDS WITH CINNAMON • 1 POINT

Put cinnamon on anything and everything. It's great for you, and it's healthily deceptive. We associate it so much with sugar that it makes us *think* we're eating something sweet and fattening even when we aren't. I put it in applesauce and on peaches. I've even had my *Biggest Loser* peeps put it in Greek yogurt with crushed almonds as a treat. Or add it to your coffee or tea as a topper.

TASTE TEST • • 2 POINTS

What are you antsy for—something salty, sweet, crunchy, or sour? Or something fat laden or decadent? If you can pinpoint what your body has a desire for, it's easier to either squelch it or satisfy it with a low-calorie option. For example, if you're craving sweet, try half a baked yam or a slice of watermelon. If you're craving crunchy, try an apple with a light spread of crunchy almond butter. If it's salt you want, try a 100-calorie bag of popchips, seaweed snacks, kale chips, or celery with low-fat ricotta cheese. (Sprinkle with a little cayenne or chili powder for extra flavor.) Popcorn alone is also a healthy, whole-grain fiber snack—the extra butter and salt that are usually added contribute the calories and bloat.

   If this kind of substitution still leaves you wanting the pizza or the brownie, remember that that's an option, too, but portion size is key. Luckily, when it comes to cravings, satisfying them doesn't take volume. Check out my next tip to see what I mean.

THIRD TIME'S A CHARM • • • 3 POINTS

As you may have gathered, I'm not big into deprivation. I'm also not into overindulgence, either. In an effort to find the middle ground, I've personally perfected my craving-management strategy. Here it is: *Take three bites.*

I'm serious. Savor three bites of whatever it is that you want, then step away from the food and distract yourself with a chore or a hobby (see my next tip). Give it 10 to 15 minutes, and chances are your craving will disappear. When you're on that third bite, you'll be thinking that you could consume the whole thing and that I (meaning me) must be an idiot. I promise, if you can muster up the willpower to wait another 15 minutes before going back for more, it's extremely likely you'll forget about wanting to do so.

As with the feeling of fullness, your body takes a beat to register the sugar and feel satisfied. Once your body knows it has gotten its fix, it's satisfied without you having to eat the entire box of cookies or the whole pint of ice cream.

GET BUSY • • 2 POINTS

When you need to distract yourself, keep busy. It's amazing how *not* hungry I am on days where I'm up to my armpits in contestant problems on the set of *Biggest Loser*. But when I work from home, I feel starved every hour. When you're busy, your mind isn't constantly searching for a way to entertain, amuse, or please itself. I want you to work at keeping busy (for some of us, that's not hard). If you aren't working, then volunteer or pursue a hobby. I don't care what you do, just keep busy. Remember, "Idle hands are the devil's playthings."

USE YOUR NOSE • 1 POINT

Aromatherapy has long been practiced as a way to curb hunger. All you have to do is dispense 1 to 3 drops of pure essential oil and inhale. I've even put it on my wrists and behind my ears like a perfume. Try these slimming scents, recommended by aromatherapists to help curb food cravings: grapefruit, cinnamon, ginger, and coriander oils.

SMELLS SO GOOD • 1 POINT

Here's another tip where your nose can help you. Dr. Alan R. Hirsch of the Smell and Taste Treatment and Research Foundation in Chicago had 3,000 volunteers sniff apples and bananas. He found that the more often they sniffed food, the less hungry they were, and the more weight they lost. His theory is that sniffing food tricks the brain into thinking you're actually eating it and as such helps to reduce appetite. I personally have experimented with using other temptation foods as a deterrent (as apples and bananas don't always float my craving boat). Although my success rate isn't 100 percent, I've been able to circumvent a brownie or two on occasion simply by smelling other sweet foods.

POLISH YOUR PEARLY WHITES •• 2 POINTS

The dentist always tells you to brush after you eat, right? Well, next time you think you're hungry, or you're ready to mindlessly binge, go brush your teeth. This quick, simple, and cheap deterrent can keep you from wreaking major havoc on your eating plan. Seriously, think about it: how good does sugar seem right after you brush your teeth? It doesn't really, right? Use this response to your advantage. I even travel with Wisps (disposable mouth fresheners that look like mini-toothbrushes), so when I'm out and about without my tooth-brush and toothpaste, I'm still covered.

ELIMINATE THE HIDDEN CULPRIT ••• 3 POINTS

Ever wonder why the food commercial says, "You can't eat just one"? It's because the manufacturer loaded that crappy food up with salt and MSG so you'll want more of it. These two ingredients are the underlying source in most foods known to cause cravings. Don't use them. Substitute lemon, lime, vinegar, onion or garlic, pepper, chili, ginger, or any other real seasonings that won't encourage your body to keep eating. Over time your taste for salt will diminish, your cravings will dissipate, you'll be less bloated, and your blood pressure will likely be lower!

Managing Stress

Excessive stress is a killer—literally. Left unchecked, stress can contribute to health problems such as obesity, high blood pressure, heart disease, and type 2 diabetes. It can sabotage your slim by wreaking havoc on your hormones—essentially throwing your body into a survival state that packs on fat and cannibalizes muscle. It also puts you in a bummer of a mood. Stress can be managed and minimized, but you have to make conscious efforts to do so.

You're probably going to want to blow off this section, because you're busy running the rat race. But I'm telling you, don't. In the long run, how you handle the excess stress in your life is going to be one of your top slimming factors, as well as the key to keeping you healthy and disease free.

CHILL OUT

GET YOUR SHUT-EYE • • • 3 POINTS

Sleep is crucial for weight loss. Getting 7 to 8 hours a night can do as much for your waistline as an actual workout. Often when I'm faced with a choice between getting 6 hours of sleep but doing a workout, and skipping the workout and sleeping 8 hours, I choose the sleep. Does that sound crazy to you coming from me? It's not— here's why.

I promised you no boring biochemistry lessons, so I'll try to make this explanation brief. Sleep has a dramatic impact on your hormone balance. You release most of your slimming hormones when you sleep, like HGH (which burns fat and maintains lean muscle mass) and leptin (which helps control and regulate appetite). Conversely, when you don't sleep, you release hormones like cortisol (which promotes fat storage) and ghrelin (which stimulates appetite). Ever had one of those days where you didn't get much sleep the night before and you feel like your stomach is a bottomless pit? Yeah, I thought so. In fact, a study from the Mayo Clinic found that shortchanging slumber by as little as 80 minutes a night leads people to take in an average of 549 more calories the next day. Prioritize your shut-eye.

Here are a few pointers to help you get your z's:

- Go to bed early.
- Don't work in bed. This habit stresses people out. Some researchers theorize that the light from our computer screens stimulates our brain and keeps us from relaxing. This leads to my next tip.
- Make sure your bedroom is dark. Leave your cell phone off or in another room; don't sleep with the TV on. Invest in black-out shades. All will help to keep your environment—and your sleep—restful.
- If you have regular trouble sleeping or staying asleep, try taking a supplement like melatonin that helps control your natural sleep-wake cycle. Or consider a product called Calm, which is a calcium magnesium blend. I swear by this combo of products and give it to all my *Biggest Loser* contestants when they're anxious and restless.
- Lighten the load. If your mind is racing, write a list of everything you need to do the next day. This always helps me feel less scattered and stressed because I've got a game plan in

place and a handle on the situation. I can go to bed feeling organized and prepared for action when I wake in the morning.

GO ON VACATION • • • 3 POINTS

Take a break. Don't fall victim to the idea that you can't unplug or be away from your work. Taking time away from your routine allows the body to replenish and repair itself. The Mind-Body Center at the University of Pittsburgh surveyed 1,399 participants recruited for studies on cardiovascular disease, breast cancer, and other conditions and found that leisure activities, including taking vacations, contributed to higher positive emotional levels and less depression among the participants. Other benefits include lower blood pressure and smaller waistlines. Women especially seem to benefit from taking vacations. According to a 2005 study conducted by Marshfield Clinic in Wisconsin, women who vacationed less frequently than once every two years were more likely to suffer from depression and increased stress than women who took vacations at least twice a year. Take your vacations. There really isn't more to say than this.

FOODS TO BUST STRESS • • 2 POINTS

Believe it or not, there are certain foods you can consume that will soothe your nerves and help keep stress hormones in check. Try to incorporate these mellowing foods into your diet as often as possible:

- **Foods rich in vitamin C.** These foods help to inhibit cortisol (aka belly-fat producing, stress-related hormone) production. Squeeze lemon into your water, put mandarin orange slices in your salad, have grapefruit with your eggs for breakfast, make a berry smoothie, have blueberries in your oatmeal. Tomatoes, melon, guava, bell pepper, kiwi, and cherries are also great options.

- **Folic acid and B vitamins.** These substances are key to producing the feel-good hormone serotonin. Be sure to eat foods rich in both of these uplifting nutrients as often as possible.
    - ✓ Folic acid is found in dark leafy greens, asparagus, broccoli, beans and lentils, avocado, sunflower seeds, okra, and brussels sprouts.
    - ✓ Vitamins B_3, B_6, and B_{12} are found in whitefish, shellfish, mussels, clams, beef, crab, poultry, and eggs.
- **Magnesium.** A deficiency in magnesium is associated with feeling low and having a poor response to stress.
    - ✓ Magnesium-rich foods are almonds, squash, and pumpkin seeds.

TRY A TONIC • 1 POINT

For those of you who don't know, homeopathy is a system of medicine that's based on the doctrine "like cures like." Essentially, homeopathic practitioners believe that a substance that causes the symptoms of a disease in healthy people will cure that disease in sick people by triggering the body's natural system of healing. While many in modern medicine say it's quackery, many others swear by it. My thoughts: if there's research that supports it—and there is—what's the harm of trying it? A study at Duke University in Durham, North Carolina, found homeopathy effective in helping to quell stress and treat anxiety disorders.

Look for stress formulas such as Nerve Tonic (from Hyland) or Sedalia (from Boiron) in your health-food store and follow the directions carefully—this is very important when using homeopathics. Many stores that sell homeopathics have salespeople who have had training in recommending remedies, so be sure to ask. Better yet, if you have the money, consult a licensed homeopath. To find one near you, contact the National Center for Homeopathy at www.healthy.net.

SAY CHEESE • 1 POINT

Smiling is a two-way mechanism. We smile when we're relaxed and happy, but smiling can also make us *feel* relaxed and happy. It's a bit of a chicken-and-egg scenario. Smiling transmits nerve impulses from the facial muscles to the limbic system, a key emotional center in the brain, tilting the neurochemical balance toward calm. That's fancy scientist talk. Just smile, as often as possible. Obviously I don't want you to cloak your emotions or fake your feelings. But when you're in a neutral head space (meaning you're not mad, not happy, and not sad), make an effort to shift your mood with a grin. It will only boost your state of mind and lift the mood of those around you.

LAUGH YOUR ASS OFF—LITERALLY • • 2 POINTS

I'm sure you've heard the phrase "Laughter is the best medicine." Considering all the positive effects laughter has on our bodies, it's daily becoming more evident how true a statement this really is. Laughter is a top stress antidote. Over the short term, it can induce physical changes in your body that stimulate circulation to the heart, lungs, and muscles; it also triggers muscle relaxation to help destress you. Laughter reduces the level of fattening stress hormones like cortisol and epinephrine (adrenaline), while simultaneously increasing levels of stress-busting hormones like endorphins and neurotransmitters. Laughter has been found to benefit the way blood flows around the body, reducing potential risk of heart disease. Corresponding research suggests that 15 minutes of daily, hearty laughter is just as important for your heart as 30 minutes of exercise 3 times a week. Over the long term, a daily laugh or two can boost your immune system, decrease your blood sugar levels, and help you sleep.

And here's the bonus: laughing burns calories. Think of a good laugh session as a spontaneous workout. Maciej Buchowski, a researcher from Vanderbilt University, found from his caloric-expenditure study that you burn 50 calories by laughing for 10 to 15 minutes. Beyond being great for your weight and health, laughing just feels good. Research has proven that people who watch funny films, which cause them to laugh out loud, experience an increase in blood flow and heart rate and a massive jump in endorphins.

Whenever you need to tickle your funny bone, go see a funny movie or rewatch your favorites. I always go back to *There's Something About Mary, Liar Liar,* and *When Harry Met Sally.* Go see a stand-up comic whom you love. Eddie Izzard and Ellen DeGeneres do it for me every time. And socialize more with your funniest friends. I've cultivated a cast of characters in my life who keep me in stiches on a regular basis. If all else fails, try joining a Laughter Yoga club. Dr. Madan Kataria, a physican from Mumbai, created the novel idea of combining unconditional laughter with yogic breathing. You'll feel so ridiculous, I guarantee you won't be able to help but crack up. There are now more than six thousand Laughter Yoga clubs in about sixty countries. Clubs are free and run by volunteers. To find one near you, log on to www.laughteryoga.org.

BE AFFIRMATIVE • 1 POINT

We talked in Chapter 5 about creating mantras, changing your vernacular, and "flipping the script," and now, yes, I'm going Stuart Smalley on you and asking you to do affirmations. Cheesy as they may be, affirmations are a good way to silence your internal critic—you know, that voice in your head that beats you up, thinks the worst, and really stresses you out. These inner monologues can have a tremendous negative effect on our lives. Creating short, positive statements will challenge, undermine, and replace these negative beliefs with a healthy, optimistic attitude that steers you toward success. The next time you feel as if your life is one disaster after another, repeat 10 times, "Everything will be okay. I can handle this."

Remember, thoughts are *things* with dynamic power. Use them to your advantage.

JUST SAY NO • • • 3 POINTS

Trying to please everyone is a surefire way to get seriously over-whelmed and stressed out. It's perfectly acceptable to have limits, and frankly, you should have them. You don't have to be everyone's hero to have value in their eyes or in the eyes of the world. Every single *Biggest Loser* contestant I've ever had tells me they took care of their entire family as a kid and that they continue to be everyone else's caretaker as adults. Obviously, it hasn't served them well—if anything, it has played a huge role in their self-neglect. Learn to say no. I get that it may make you feel really uncomfortable and that you think it's nearly impossible, but once you go out on a limb and try it, you'll see that the world won't end. Quite the contrary, you'll probably feel great, having made a little time for yourself for a change. I know I always get resentful when I commit to things at my own expense—miss my workouts or lose sleep because of an overly packed schedule. Screw that. Here are two simple tips to help you break the "Just say no" ice:

1. Be sympathetic but firm. This gives the person the signal that you care but won't cave to pressure. You're showing that you won't change your mind. Simply say "I'm sorry. I'd love to help, but I'm just swamped right now."

2. You don't owe an explanation—less is more. "I'm crazy busy. Wish I could but I can't." Keep it that simple. We build up too many barri-ers in our minds about saying no.

Remember, saying no doesn't mean you're being disagreeable, causing conflict, burning a bridge, or being rude. It simply means you don't have the time. Say it nicely and respectfully, and all will work out fine.

BREATHE IT IN • 1 POINT

Play with aromatherapy again, but this time use it for relaxation purposes. The following essential oils are all soothing: anise, basil, bay, chamomile, eucalyptus, lavender, rose, and thyme. Choose one you love, and place it in a little tray by your bedside, on your desk, or even on your temples for an instant calming effect.

GET HORIZONTAL • • • 3 POINTS

If sex has been at the bottom of your to-do list for too long, move it to the top. Sex improves every aspect of your life—emotional, mental, and physical.

Doing "the dirty" boosts confidence, improves intimacy, and increases levels of endorphins, those mood-boosting chemicals in the brain. It's flat out one of the best total-body relaxers. It will raise your heartbeat to aerobic levels and burn an average of 200 calories during a 30-minute "session." This translates into losing about a pound for every 17.5 times you have sex. Not too shabby. Researchers report that sex reduces food cravings and stimulates chemicals in the body that help control appetite, subsequently facilitating your ability to reduce calorie intake. And depending upon your positions and routine, you can build muscle from frequent sex. I think listing positions here, with corresponding muscle groups, would be going a bit overboard (although I actually considered it). Just use your imagination and get creative; I bet you can get a total-body workout in as a bonus to great sex. So what are you waiting for? Get busy.

GET A NEW BEST FRIEND • • 2 POINTS

You don't have to jettison your old best friend, but studies show that owning a pet can help you lose weight, lower blood pressure, and reduce stress levels. These are not small side effects but rather dramatic ones. For each of these issues, pets may be even better than drugs. (This is probably why I have three dogs, two horses, and a bird.) A study at the University of Buffalo compared two groups of hypertensive New York stockbrokers: one group had no pets, while the other group took in dogs or cats after being petless for five years. Those with pets were found to have lower blood pressure and heart rates than those without. The researcher seemed to find that the drugs normally used to control and reduce blood pressure weren't quite as effective as animals. (The great part about this story is that many in the petless group went out and got pets after they heard the results.)

Another study, conducted at the University of Missouri at Columbia, discovered that obese, sedentary individuals who walked a dog—their own or one they borrowed—for 20 minutes 5 days a week, lost more weight than those who walked alone. They lost 14 more pounds per person over a one-year period without even dieting. And one more: researchers at the University of Victoria in British Columbia found that of 351 participants, those who owned dogs walked, on average, 300 minutes per week, while nondog owners walked only 168 minutes a week.

Okay, this is probably more research than you ever wanted to hear, and I'm sorry to bombard you, but I'm pretty passionate about this one. If you already own a pet—a dog or otherwise—you already know you can't live without it. If you don't, consider *adopting* one. You'll be saving a life, and it can do miracles for your health, mental state, and waistline.

SAY OMMMM • 1 POINT

Meditation has been shown to have a wealth of health benefits, and it can calm your mind and reduce your stress. It requires you to tap all the self-regulation systems and self-monitoring mechanisms in your brain—the prefrontal cortex (which helps you make smart choices) and the anterior cingulate cortex (which helps you become aware of when you're making these choices and when you aren't). The more you activate these systems, the stronger they will become and the less impulsive and calmer you will become. Regular meditation allows you to literally build your willpower.

Here's a simple exercise: Meditate for 5 minutes every day this week. What does that mean exactly? Just sit quietly with your eyes closed and focus on your breathing. Inhale as deeply as possible in and out through your nose. Feel your breath fill your lungs and expand your belly on the inhale, then deflate like a balloon on the exhale. While 5 minutes of this might seem like an eternity at first, fight your way through it. Your brain will want to wander. That's okay—just pull it back to your breath when it does. It's amazing how much more relaxed you will feel when it's over. It gets easier every time you do it.

LISTEN TO THE BEATLES—*ASK FOR HELP!* • • • 3 POINTS

Americans pride themselves on being mavericks, but this attitude hasn't truly served us well. Researchers expect that 75 percent of Americans will be obese by 2030, and cancer and heart disease are on the rise, so we clearly as a nation need to come up with something that will help. Granted, our problems won't all go away if we simply ask for help. But working together on them will surely help minimize them. We are social creatures who work best in groups where we cooperate and collaborate with each other and appreciate each other's unique knowledge and strengths. We *all* need help from time to time. Those of us who reap the spoils are those who feel worthy and secure enough to ask for it.

If you're stressed about finding a job, ask your social circle to put feelers out to help you network. If you're struggling with your diet and/or fitness regimen and are not getting the results you want, ask someone who is knowledgeable in those areas, or who has lost weight themselves, for information and advice that might point you in the right direction. If you're intimidated by the thought of going to the gym, ask your significant other or best friend to go with you, so you don't feel so uncomfortable.

A little help goes a long way. People may not always be able to accommodate you, but if you don't ask, you don't get. Even if you get what you need from your support network only half the time, it can make an enormous difference in helping you live the slim and narrow.

....

"It's Not in My Budget"

People often use a lack of money as an excuse to not get healthy, blaming budgetary restrictions for their expanding waistlines. I would argue that buying cheap food now will cost you a fortune in health care costs down the road (truly, as I mentioned previously, medical issues are the number-one cause of bankruptcy in our country), but I'm not insensitive to the immediate issue of affordability. Here are some tips you can follow to fatten your bank account while slimming your physique. Note: I'm not assigning these tips points, as they don't directly affect your slim. The one exception is "Be fitness frugal," which affects your ability to exercise *and* to be cost-effective. You don't need to clip coupons to be slim, but if budget restraints are an obstacle for you, this section is your go-to for overcoming them.

BE FOOD FRUGAL

CATCH A CHILL

I always tell you to buy fresh, but there's one exception to this rule: you can purchase fruits and veggies that are flash frozen. Not only will it be more cost effective, but the frozen versions may actually have more nutrients (because they're frozen before their nutrients have a chance to oxidize). Remember, fruits and veggies age like we do, and the longer they ripen, the more vitamins and minerals they lose.

SHOP THE BINS

Buy grains, beans, nuts, spices, and cereals from bulk bins. Many supermarkets have them, and it will save you money because you won't be paying the food companies' packaging costs. (It's also good for the environment.) Some of the best bin bargains are grains and legumes. A recent study compared bins to major store brands and found that long-grain brown rice was a dollar cheaper per pound in bulk than in a package. Lentils were 80 cents cheaper in the bin. Bulk black beans cost 99 cents per pound, while the packaged version cost $2.19. Oatmeal's a bin bargain at 69 cents per pound, compared to $2.92 if you opt for a name brand. Plus, you can buy as much or as little as you want, because you control the exact quantity purchased.

BULK UP

Stores like Costco can offer their products at a discount because they purchase and sell in bulk. The only issue is that perishable foods might go to waste if you aren't planning on eating 20 chicken breasts or 5 pounds of apples. The solution is simple: freeze proteins, then defrost them when you're ready to eat them. For fruits and veggies, try splitting them with a friend. Literally split the cost and the product, so you'll get the amount you need with no waste and at a discount.

BE GENERIC

Don't be sucked in by expensive marketing campaigns for name brands. Generic and store-brand products are cheaper than their name-brand equivalents and are usually of similar quality. This is because you aren't paying the profit margin of a third party (the name-brand company).

BE THRIFTY

Clip coupons. In the past, coupons for organics and healthier foods were hard to come by, but that's changing. Now that many big-box stores like Safeway and Walmart are starting their own organic food lines, coupons are more readily available. Here's a great website dedicated to saving you money when shopping organic: www.organicgrocerydeals.com. You can go to the website for your favorite products. More often than not it offers discount codes and coupons you can print out and take to the market with you.

SLIM MYTH:
Iceberg lettuce is just as healthy as other greens.

FAST FACT: Iceberg lettuce is made up of 95 percent water and contains only small amounts of fiber, vitamins, and minerals compared to other dark, leafy greens. Try switching to arugula, spinach, kale, or romaine to get the best nutrient boost possible out of your salad. The darker the lettuce, the more nutritious it is.

VISIT NEARBY FARMER'S MARKETS

Because farmer's markets involve minimal if any costs for transport, packaging, and advertising, because the food is direct from farm to table, you automatically pay less. Organic food at the farmer's market may be more expensive than nonorganics at a traditional supermarket, but it will still be cheaper than buying organics at a supermarket.

GROW YOUR OWN

This is an obvious one. You can produce up to 100 pounds of food a year in a six-foot-square raised bed in your backyard. I know because we do it at my house. The food you raise is all natural and nearly free. While this might seem daunting, it really isn't that hard. Here are a few websites to get you started:

www.organicgardening.com
www.smilinggardener.com
www.organicgardeningtips.com

For those of you who are going to bitch at me about the weather where you live, you can always jar and can your crops for the off seasons.

GO SURFING

Healthy, slimming foods are often cheaper online because you're not paying for a market's expensive storefront. The GreenPeople directory from the Organic Consumer Association (www.organic consumers.org/purelink.html) is a good place to begin your online search for affordable foods. And be sure to check out the list of cyber-markets offering organic products in your area at www.organic kitchen.com. By the way, it doesn't have to be an organic grocer. Even Amazon now allows you to do your marketing online for a cheaper price.

PAY CASH

Studies show that we tend to spend and even buy less when we pay for our goods (in particular junk food) with cash. A study out of Cornell University, published in the *Journal of Consumer Research*, found that both the cash and credit card groups spent about the same amount on "healthy" staples like oatmeal, fat-free yogurt, and the like. But the cash group spent 42 percent more on junk food when they used a credit card. Cut up those credit cards, baby! Or if that's too drastic, try this trick—I used it when I was younger: I froze my credit cards in a bowl of water. This way when there was an emergency and I actually needed them, they were there, but it tremendously reduced my ability to overspend and impulse-buy because I paid with my hard-earned dollars.

BUY A SHARE IN A COMMUNITY-SUPPORTED AGRICULTURE PROGRAM (CSA)

When you buy a share in a CSA, you pay a portion of a local farm's operating expenses. In return, you receive a weekly box of fresh fruit and vegetables, at a cost of about $300 to $500 for a 24-to-26-week growing season. Many CSAs accept monthly payments, and you may be able to buy a half-share if a full one is too costly. Some folks save even more money by actually helping out on the farm every now and then. To find a CSA near you, check the websites of government and nonprofit organizations such as the Alternative Farming Systems Information Center (afsic.nal.usda.gov); Food Routes (www.foodroutes.org); and Local Harvest (www.localharvest.org).

JOIN A FOOD CO-OP

A food cooperative is a member-owned business that provides groceries and other products to its members at a discount. Most of the products are organic and come from local family farms. All you do is sign up and pay some dues. Co-op members who volunteer to work may get additional discounts on any products they buy. To find a co-op near you, check out the food co-op directory on the website of the online magazine *Cooperative Grocer* (www.cooperativegrocer.coop/coops). If there's no co-op in your area and you've got the time and desire to do so, you can start your own. Cooperative Grocer Network (www.cgin.coop) has a brochure to show you how.

JOIN A BUYING CLUB

Buying club members purchase food and other slimming products in bulk and then split the stash—and you can get as much as 30 to 40 percent off retail this way. Ask a co-op near you about starting a buying club with your friends and neighbors. Or ask a local natural food store where they get their goods, then contact the distributor directly.

COMPARISON SHOP

There are many resources and places for buying healthy food. See how they compare pricewise. For example, in some areas, organic milk at Trader Joe's is nearly $2 cheaper than similar organic milk sold at Whole Foods. Our organic baby food is $15 cheaper at Ralph's than at our local organic grocery store. Do your homework before you shop, and see who offers the best deals.

CUT THE CRAP

I'm willing to bet you buy *at least* $20 worth of crap a week that you don't need, which you can and should rechannel into healthy, slimming food. It's time to evaluate your weekly spending habits and kick the nonessentials to the curb. For example:

1. How much are you spending on gossip rags and magazines weekly? These are like three to five bucks a pop. Read this stuff online. It's free.

2. How many times do you hit the coffee shop every week? Beverages cost anywhere from $2 to $5 each there. If you spend $2.75 on a cup of joe every day, it will cost you $715 a year. That's $14 a week that could go toward healthier food. Make your coffee at home or work. Save the cash for something that will contribute to your new slim lifestyle.

3. Remember my "Beverage Basics" discussion in Chapter 1, on healthy liquid consumption? Stop wasting money on bottled water, juices, and sodas. These are nonessentials, and adding insult to injury, most of them make you fat.

4. Don't be lazy. Walk or bike wherever you're going. This will save you money on fuel, public transport, and even parking. The average car owner actually spends a thousand dollars on parking a year. At

the very least, self-park and walk to your destination from there. And the extra mileage you log walking only furthers your slim aspirations.

5. Nonbank ATM fees can really add up. It can cost $2 to $4.50 to withdraw as little as $20. Once a week go to your bank and withdraw the amount you need to get you through, so your bank account won't get hammered left and right with unnecessary fees.

I could really go on and on with this information, but ultimately the onus is going to fall on you to take a good hard look at where you financially hemorrhage cash. Stop the bleeding, and proactively redirect some of it toward your health. As I've told you, sickness and obesity are expensive. Slim people use far fewer medications, if any. They require medical attention far less often, other than routine check-ups. They don't get debilitating, life-threatening, bankrupting sicknesses like heart disease or cancer nearly as often as those who are obese.

BE FITNESS FRUGAL

ACCEPT HAND-ME-DOWNS • 1 POINT
Scoop up used DVDs or fitness equipment for a steal. Amazon.com is a great resource for these products.

HIRE A PRO—ONCE • 1 POINT
I touched on this in Chapter 5 with the "Ask for feedback" tip, but it has a slightly different meaning here. The goal now is to save money. Buying one session with a trainer can go a long way to that end. Investing in the expertise one time saves you from wasting money elsewhere on fitness products you don't need.

GET MOVED • 1 POINT

I discussed exercising in Chapter 2. Not only is using your own body weight convenient and healthy—it's *free*! See Chapter 2 for tips on bodyweight exercises that you can do to get a killer workout at no cost. Plus, you can always get outside and go hiking, run up some stairs, or pound the pavement for a jog.

....

Fitting Workouts in with Kids

I love my kids more than anyone and anything on the planet, but let's face facts: staying slim with young kids in your life can be difficult. The following are tips and tricks I've had to put into practice since my son and daughter came into my life.

WITH 'EM

PRACTICE TOGETHERNESS •• 2 POINTS

If you have kids, exercise with them. If they're little, put them in a jogging stroller and go for a run, toss them in a sidecar and go for a bike ride, or pop them into a baby carrier and go for a hike. I've even put my daughter on my paddleboard (in a life vest, of course) and gone paddleboarding. Your kids will love spending this time together, you're setting a positive example for them early on, and you're getting your burn in.

PLAY • 1 POINT

Ever chased a toddler around in a game of tag or hide and seek? Ever hit the playground with them? It'll wear you out and burn some calories. If your kids are a bit older, play games with them.

FAST FACT: Ice or cold water is the way to go when you're trying to minimize muscle soreness. When you exercise, your blood vessels open wider and stay that way for at least an hour afterward. Soreness occurs when waste products like lactic acid settle into your muscles through these dilated vessels. Colder temps constrict vessels, limiting the amount of waste that accumulates.

Shoot hoops, play catch, ride bikes, go Rollerblading. You know I believe in playtime for you—now make it a family affair. They'll have a blast, and you'll be amazed at how much stress and steam you'll let off while you're getting your workout in.

THERE'S NO PLACE LIKE HOME
• • • 3 POINTS

While we talked earlier about the value of having a DVD fitness library, it won't be of help to you unless you use it—which with the little ones around can be challenging. Try making the kids a part of your workout. I can't tell you how many moms send me cute pictures of their toddlers barking orders at them while they use my workout videos. The kids think it's hilarious, and you'll get your burn on—it's a win-win.

TAKE THEM WITH YOU • • • 3 POINTS

Join a gym with a childcare service or room. They can play while you pump some iron and take care of you. Most gyms offer something—take advantage of it.

WITHOUT 'EM

MULTITASK • 1 POINT

Answer e-mails on the StairMaster. Do conference calls from the elliptical. Read a business document on the stationary bike. You get the idea. While this is the last thing I want to see you do (my goal is for you to train with intensity and focus for optimal results), there are days when I've had no choice but to do it. It's likely the same for you. This advice falls under the cliché that doing something is better than doing nothing.

MAKE THE TRADE-OFF • • • 3 POINTS

If you have a significant other, take turns watching the kids. This tip works really well for Heidi and me, plus it allows each of us to grab a minute of sanity and often much-needed alone time. She'll go do yoga while I take the kids, then later that night or the next day I'll go for a bike ride or a jog while she watches them. If you don't have a significant other, try a friend. Do a sitting swap, and spread the good health.

CALL GRANDMA • • • 3 POINTS

You know who loves your kids as much as you? *Your parents!* This is why God gave us grandparents. Seriously. If you have parents or family in the area, ask them to watch the kids once a week while you get your workout in. They get their bonding time in, you get pumped, and everybody feels good. I'm lucky my mom is always up to a Sunday afternoon. Thank God.

BE SNEAKY • • • 3 POINTS

Get up early, and exercise while they sleep. This is one I will never adhere to, but for you morning people, it works like a charm. Simply pop in a workout video and go to town. Or if you have home equipment and can give yourself a great workout, go for it. If morning isn't your best time, as for me, you can also get it in after they go to sleep. I've done that, and it works pretty well. I put the kids to bed around seven, pop in my workout video, get my sweat on, and then eat dinner. It's not my favorite solution, but it's an option for those days when nothing else will work, and it helps me piece together my 4 to 5 weekly workouts.

....

Tick-tock: Overcoming Time Constraints

Another excuse people use for not eating right or working out is time. You already have the answers to this problem, as I've made sure to sprinkle them throughout *Slim for Life*—you may have noticed that many of the tips are multipurpose. To not be painfully repetitive, let me just highlight the tricks to overcoming time issues that make this excuse totally invalid. By the way, you get no extra points for using these repeat tips; you've already counted your points and been rewarded in other chapters for squeezing your workout in and grabbing healthy food in a hurry.

CATCH A BURN ON THE RUN

1. Work out on your lunch hour.

2. Build a home gym or use DVDs to fit in a quick 30-minute burn session before or after work.

3. Use the NEAT tips from pages 96 and 126.

4. Work out at your desk, and be sure to stand up and pace while on the phone.

5. If you have kids, work out with them or ask a friend or family member to watch them a few times a week so you can get your burn on.

6. Schedule your workout using whatever method works best for you—a day timer, your phone alarm. Treat it with importance, as you would any other appointment.

7. Exercise during commercial breaks for your favorite TV shows (although if you have time to watch TV, you *do* have time for a proper workout!).

8. Be a weekend warrior and get it in on Saturday and Sunday.

EAT HEALTHY IN A HURRY

1. Pack your lunch.

2. Bring healthy snacks with you at all times. (You can even invest in a small cooler or cold pack. There are no excuses here!)

3. Enter your go-to restaurant's contact info in your phone or write it on an accessible list. That way you can grab a slimming meal on the run. Just call ahead and order so you can take out a healthy meal.

4. Modify your food order when eating out to create the healthiest meal from a restaurant's options.

....

Access Denied?

As with time constraints, I've also addressed the access issue previously throughout this book, but in case you didn't catch the dual benefits of those bits of advice, I'll give you a quick refresher so you can put two and two together. (Note: If you think you're getting points for these tips, nope; that'd be "double-dipping." As with the tips for overcoming time constraints, we've already assigned them and added them up in earlier chapters.)

FITNESS

1. Build a home gym.

2. Use your local environment, from running and hiking trails to the stairs in your apartment building, home, or hotel.

3. Bring DVDs and exercise tubing with you on the road, so even if there isn't a gym near you, you're covered.

4. Don't let poor outdoor weather conditions deter you from working out. It's an excuse that has no legs—literally. If you're an avid outdoor exerciser, try these workout alternatives so you stay fit during the winter months as well as avoid winter weight gain.

✓ Walk in the mall, or purchase a winter pass at a local gym until you can go back outside.

✓ Take your swimming indoors, and vary how you use the pool. Invest in a deep-water buoyancy belt for deep-water running; this is one of the most challenging workouts you'll ever do. It's great for cross-training, too; you can find out more at www.aquajogger.com or www .splashinternational.biz.

SLIM MYTH:

Working out on an empty stomach burns more fat.

FAST FACT: Don't exercise on an empty stomach. If you do, you'll have considerably less energy for your workout and you run the risk of cannibalizing your own muscle tissue. You see, your body needs a certain amount of sugar for fuel when training. When you don't have available blood sugar or stored sugar in your muscles, your body will convert your own muscle tissue into energy. Plus, the harder you train, the more calories and fat you'll burn, and if you haven't eaten, you probably won't have a very intense workout. Get yourself a little snack about an hour before you work out—something with carbs and protein like a whey shake, or an apple with almond butter.

✓ Strap on snowshoes (not that I have ever done this, or know anyone who has, but rumor has it this is a killer workout) or cross-country skis (far more realistic) for a kickass lower-body and cardio workout—you'll burn approximately 263 more calories in 30 minutes (based on a 145-pound female). Find out more at www .caloriesperhour.com.

FOOD

1. Shop for healthy food online. Every supermarket chain is offering this now, from Whole Foods to Vons. In fact, even Walmart and Amazon have this service.

2. Remember to look for the cheese stick, the hard-boiled egg, the healthy energy bar, and the nut options at convenience stores—if that's your only option when out and about.

3. At fattening restaurants, pick the healthiest choices, and modify the dishes to fit your slim needs.

4. When you're traveling, scout the area where you're going online, or use the "Places" locator on your phone—this nifty GPS tool (comes free on iPhones and most Androids) identifies your location on the spot. Then it will give you information about restaurants,

> **EZ CALORIE CUT**
>
> Instead of ordering your ice cream in a waffle cone, have it in a cup. **CUT: 121 CALORIES**

cafés, coffee places, and the like so you know the food choices that surround you. This modern technology is very cool—there's absolutely *no* excuse to say "I have no idea where to get healthy food."

Busting Through Plateaus

I bet you've been waiting for me to address this bad boy of an issue all chapter long. Well, here goes. I actually don't believe in the idea of a plateau. Why? Because in my experience 90 percent of the time if a person has supposedly hit one, it's because he or she is simply eating too much and not keeping track of calories. Or they've been slacking off in the intensity, frequency, or both, of their workouts. There is one *rare* and real occasion where plateauing is real. Here it is: if you have lost a good amount of weight, your energy intake has significantly slowed, and your energy expenditure has increased due to exercise, your body can panic and throw on the brakes. Biologically, your body can think it's approaching a phase of famine and will automatically release hormones to slow down your weight loss for survival purposes. Here are the best ways to rectify the problem ASAP.

FINE-TUNE YOUR PROGRESS

INVESTIGATE • • • 3 POINTS

Open up a notebook and write down what you eat for three days. See if you have unintentionally let your calories slip and you're eating too much. If so, the fix is simple: rein it in a bit.

UP YOUR CALORIES • • • 3 POINTS

If you've done proper investigating, you aren't overeating, and you've plateaued, then you need to actually *increase* your calories. Here's what to do: start the next week with one high-calorie day at an intake of 2,000 calories. Then for the subsequent six days, increase your previous calorie intake by 10 percent. So if you were eating 1,200 calories when you plateaued, then for the next six days after your high-calorie day, eat 1,320 calories per day. This will reassure your body that you're not starving, and it will go back into fat-burning mode. I know the idea of upping your calories will probably freak you out, but I'm a master at this. And even if I'm wrong (which I'm not), you'll only be taking in an additional 1,700 calories over the course of the week. That's about half a pound. So take a deep breath, relax, and do what I say.

DON'T OVERDO IT • • • 3 POINTS

This tip applies only to those of you with 10 or fewer pounds to lose. Oftentimes you animals go too far and end up eating too little and working out too hard. Buddy, you have to understand that losing vanity pounds versus losing unhealthy weight are two completely different things from a biological perspective. Your body wants to shed weight when it's obese. But if you want to be a size 2 instead of a 6, your body is likely not going to be on board with it. This is because you're still healthy with a little "meat on your bones" (and I do mean little). From an evolutionary perspective, this is an ideal state for your body in the event of a famine. Yes, you and I know that's not at all likely to happen here in America, but your body and your genes haven't caught up to modern times yet. The key is to create no more than a 750-to-800-calorie deficit a day *maximum*. For example, if you burn 2,500 calories total in a day, then don't eat fewer than 1,700 calories. If you're not sure how to figure out what your active metabolic rate is, go back to "Live in the red" in Chapter 1. This way your body won't panic, think it's starving, and switch to fat-storage mode.

MIX IT UP • • • 3 POINTS

If you're in a rut at the gym and have been doing the same things for weeks, change up your routine. Remember, your body is a very efficient machine. It adapts to external stimuli very quickly. As you get fitter, a workout that used to require a ton of energy to perform may now require much less; your body has adapted and become adept at doing it. Don't forget you must change your routine at least every two weeks, so that it's not routine to your body.

TWEAK YOUR DIAL • • • 3 POINTS

This one is a bit tricky, because I have to leave you to your own devices a bit. You're going to gauge the direction to turn your exercise intensity dial. You might need to turn it up, by getting in more days, or conversely turn it down by taking a couple days off. Here's how you know. If you're working out hard and noticing frequent feelings of fatigue as well as a decrease in your exercise performance at the gym, you're overdoing it and need a few days off. (By the way, this shouldn't happen to you if you follow the specifics I laid out in Chapter 2.) On the other hand, if you've been doing the same resistance exercises, maintaining the same cardio intensity, and not really feeling winded or sore after your workouts, you need to kick your butt into gear and step it up a notch. Run faster, lift more, do your push-ups on your hands and feet instead of your hands and knees. Got me? Good!

ADD IT UP, DROP IT OFF

GIVE YOURSELF 3 POINTS

- [ ] Think it through.
- [ ] Take inventory.
- [ ] Check for thirst.
- [ ] Shout it from the mountaintops.
- [ ] Eat for free.
- [ ] Remember the rules.
- [ ] Out of sight—out of mind.
- [ ] Have an emergency plan.
- [ ] Play a zero-sum game.
- [ ] Third time's a charm.
- [ ] Eliminate the hidden culprit.
- [ ] Get your shut-eye.
- [ ] Go on vacation.
- [ ] Just say no.
- [ ] Get horizontal.
- [ ] Listen to the Beatles—*ask for help!*
- [ ] There's no place like home.
- [ ] Take them with you.
- [ ] Make the trade-off.
- [ ] Call Grandma.
- [ ] Be sneaky.
- [ ] Investigate.
- [ ] Up your calories.
- [ ] Don't overdo it.
- [ ] Mix it up.
- [ ] Tweak your dial.

GIVE YOURSELF 2 POINTS

- [ ] Slow your roll.
- [ ] Pound the pavement.
- [ ] Start with soup.
- [ ] Taste test.
- [ ] Get busy.
- [ ] Polish your pearly whites.
- [ ] Foods to bust stress.
- [ ] Laugh your ass off—literally.
- [ ] Get a new best friend.
- [ ] Practice togetherness.

GIVE YOURSELF 1 POINT

- [ ] Bust a mood.
- [ ] Be a little nutty.
- [ ] Keep it cool.
- [ ] TiVo it.
- [ ] Heat it up.
- [ ] Practice yoga.
- [ ] Engage in teatime.
- [ ] Psych out your taste buds with cinnamon.
- [ ] Use your nose.
- [ ] Smells so good.
- [ ] Try a tonic.
- [ ] Say cheese.
- [ ] Be affirmative.

☐ Breathe it in.

☐ Say ommmm.

☐ Accept hand-me-downs.

☐ Hire a pro—once.

☐ Get moved.

☐ Play.

☐ Multitask.

_____ **Total *points* for Chapter 6**

_____ **Total number of *tips* I'm incorporating**

CHAPTER 7

SUPERCHARGE YOUR SLIM

This chapter will tell you about extremely novel ways to eat, move, and even dress to get and look slimmer! Most of what you'll find here are obscure ideas, and some may even sound absurd, but all of them are safe, and all of them work. I promise! (You'll also find a few more general tips that didn't fall neatly into the other chapters. I put them here so you'll have even more tools in your slim arsenal.)

The point of this chapter is to give you an edge—period. My whole life I've looked for ways to beat the status quo: not because I'm a rebel trying to reinvent the wheel, but because I'd rather think of myself as a visionary (aka extremely impatient individual) who is looking for faster, more effective ways to work and transform the human body. While it's true that new research comes out every day, I feel confident that I've covered every cutting-edge, off-the-radar, supercharged, slimming shortcut imaginable in this book, with this chapter as a grand finale.

We'll start with some basics and then travel off the beaten path into the newer, rarer, cutting-edge info. Enjoy supercharging.

The Slim Life

SLIM SAVVY SECRETS

DON'T BE A PARTY ANIMAL • • • 3 POINTS

Seriously. Grow up and leave it at the frat house. Drugs, cigarettes, and excessive drinking—none are hot. Tragic is more like it. And on top of that, heavy partying wreaks absolute havoc on your health and your metabolism. Just say no. Get high on life.

MAKE A DATE WITH YOUR SCALE • • • 3 POINTS

The scale can be most folks' worst nightmare, rightfully so. It's often abused or misused, and it's capable of delivering really crappy news. That said, when used correctly, the scale can be one of your most valuable weight-loss tools. Think of it as a compass. It simply lets you know when you're on track and doing things right, or off track and in need of a course correction.

Here's what not to do: do *not* get on the scale every day. Your weight is going to shift not only from day to day but at different times during a single day, due to body fluid fluctuations. You might have a pickle one night and be up a pound on the scale the next day because of all the sodium it contains. Remember, salt makes you hold water. Or maybe you haven't gone to the bathroom yet (gross, I know, but it had to be said), and that's literally weighing you down a bit.

The problem with obsessive scale

SLIM MYTH:

Losing 2 pounds a week is healthy.

FAST FACT: Losing 2 pounds a week is *realistic*, but it isn't necessarily healthier than losing 3, 4, or 5. The key to healthy weight loss is the method you use to lose it. If you're working out and eating right, then it's perfectly healthy if you lose more than 2 pounds a week.

abusers is that when the numbers on the scale fluctuate daily, it freaks them out and they get easily discouraged as well as overly anxious. The best way to use the scale is once a week, same scale, same day of the week, same time of day. If you choose Friday at nine a.m., then that's your weigh-in day and time each week. This consistency gives you a far more accurate read; by waiting a week, you'll allow time for the scale to actually show weight loss. If you follow this guideline and the scale goes up or doesn't budge from the previous week, you'll know you need to make some adjustments to your eating regimen or exercise routine. It's that simple.

STANDING ROOM ONLY • • 2 POINTS

Stand whenever and wherever you can, as an alternative to sitting. Standing burns 1.5 times more calories than sitting. Stand when you're at the doctor's office, stand when you work at your computer (I put mine on the kitchen counter), and stand when you watch TV. Just stand. In addition, some research suggests that sitting may actually speed up your body's production of fat. The theory is that when we lounge on a sofa or chair, we exert force on our fat cells, causing them to stretch out and generate even more fat. Not sure I buy that one fully, but I know that the increased calorie burn that comes from standing is a sure thing. Be sure to stay on your feet as often as possible.

FIDGET • • 2 POINTS

James Levine, M.D., of the Mayo Clinic in Rochester, Minnesota, has spent years studying the effect daily movement has on metabolism. His findings may surprise you. Though they're annoying to be around, individuals who can't stop moving, who constantly fidget, tap their feet, swing their arms, and pace burn up to 350 more calories per day than sedentary people. This difference in calorie burn can add up to nearly 37 pounds a year! The message is clear; even if you have a desk job, find a way to keep moving. When I had a desk job, I used to play with drumsticks on a drum pad. Give that one a try. It's superfun, and it made me feel cool.

LIMIT TV TIME • • • 3 POINTS

Keep TV viewing time to no more than 14 hours a week (no more than 2 hours per day). You might be thinking "duh," but just hold on for a beat and give me a little credit—there's more to it than you think. It's true that TV keeps you sedentary, but it can make you fat for another reason: as Harvard researchers report, being a couch potato boosts the effects of obesity-promoting genes. They tracked 32 genetic variants that were known to have genetic associations with BMI (body mass index) in study participants who watched 40-plus hours of TV a week. These fat-promoting variants ended up being three times more potent than those in genetically similar individuals who logged much less tube time *independent* of their physical exercise. TV rots your brain anyway; didn't your mother ever tell you that? I don't know about yours, but my mom is never wrong. Find something else to do that stimulates your body and your mind the majority of the time.

BE HOT AND COLD • 1 POINT

Turn your air conditioner and your heater down or, better yet, off, if you can stand it. I don't want you to freeze to death in the winter or get heat stroke in the summer, but I do want you to force your body to regulate its own temperature as much as possible. It burns more calories. When your body temperature changes, your heart rate increases because it's working harder trying to prevent overheating or overcooling. As a result, you burn slightly more calories. According to a 2000 study published in *Medicine and Science in Sports and Exercise*, BMR will change by 7 percent for each temperature change of 0.9 degrees Fahrenheit. The other good news is that you'll save on your electric bill!

GET IT TOGETHER •• 2 POINTS

By "getting it together," I don't necessarily mean becoming neater, cleaner, or more punctual, although those things certainly don't suck. Rather, I mean arranging the things in your life so that you open your time and space to all the great opportunities life has to offer.

Disorganization hampers you by creating chaos in your life and obstacles that make it difficult for you to jump at opportunities when they come along. Keeping your environment organized, at home and at work, can benefit your mental and physical health in any number of ways. Getting control of the clutter will allow you to do and accomplish more in your day. Honestly, how much time do you waste being scattered? Think of *all* the things you could do with that time! You could hit the gym, squeeze in some extra sleep, or spend quality time playing with your kid.

Organization also enhances self-esteem. How you maintain your living environment is a direct reflection of your relationship with yourself. If your office is a mess, you'll be distracted and unproductive at work. A messy kitchen may mean you're not giving proper attention to your own nourishment. A messy bathroom may indicate that you're neglecting your hygiene. Ultimately, the more organized, clean, and tidy you keep your life, the more you can achieve. Don't believe me? A study from Indiana University showed that people with the cleanest homes have *far* higher levels of physical activity in all aspects of their lives than those whose homes are messy and unkempt. By keeping your life and your surroundings organized and well looked after, you're buying yourself more precious time to fit in your slim agenda. And you're making a statement that you value yourself and deserve a good quality of life.

KICK-START YOUR WEEK ON THE WEEKEND • 1 POINT

Start a healthy initiative on a Saturday or Sunday. Mondays are typically chaotic for everyone. You're usually being pulled in a million directions, from work obligations to family commitments. In fact, studies show that exerting energy and self-control in one area can make it hard to exert it in another. This is why I tell you that will-power is like a muscle—the more you use it, the more fatigued it can get. So make Saturday or Sunday your set-up-for-success day. Get your hard-core workouts in on these days. Plan your work-outs for the week, do your healthy grocery shopping, and prepare a week's worth of healthy food so you can grab and go when time is scarce on Monday through Friday.

> **EZ CALORIE CUT**
> Instead of 6 ounces of french fries, eat a 6-ounce baked potato. **CUT: 400 CALORIES**

WEIRD FOOD AND FITNESS TIPS THAT WORK

BE MINTY FRESH • 1 POINT

This one is cool, literally. A study conducted at Wheeling Jesuit University found that the smell of peppermint can help you work out harder and faster, upping your calorie burn by as much as 15 percent. Athletes who sniffed mint gripped harder, ran faster, and pushed more weight. I dab a couple drops of essential peppermint oil on my neck or wrists before my workout, and then I go to town.

COLD HANDS, KILLER WORKOUT • 1 POINT

The key to a longer workout may be right in the palm of your hand. A recent study from Stanford University found that women who cooled off their hands while on the treadmill outlasted their hot-handed counterparts by more than 8 minutes. Another study revealed that women who wore a cooling glove during exercise for 12 weeks increased their walking speed, decreased their blood pressure, and lost 3 more inches from their waistline than those who didn't. Chilling your hands sends colder blood back to your heart, helping to cool your core temperature, which decreases fatigue while boosting endurance. You can try the Cool Point Hand Cooler for approximately $20 at www.amazon.com. Another option is to simply bring an ice-cold water bottle with you to the gym and hold it in your hands. Taking icy swigs every 10 minutes can also help to douse your body heat. Last, consider walking or jogging in cold weather without your gloves.

TREAD WISELY • • 2 POINTS

Research suggests that you may unknowingly run more slowly on a treadmill than you would run outside. When people were asked to pick a pace on the treadmill equivalent to their typical outdoor pace, they selected a speed that was 27 percent lower than their actual outdoor pace. This is because the treadmill lacks "backward optic flow"—the perception of movement as you pass objects or people. So instead of gauging your intensity arbitrarily, gauge it by heart rate. Check your heart rate when you run outdoors and make sure when you run on the treadmill that it matches.

BE A ROCK 'N' ROLLER • 1 POINT

The next time you have one of those "I'm gonna be sore for days" workouts, consider getting a quick massage right after the work-out. Researchers put 11 young, healthy men through a strenuous workout, then immediately gave them 10 minutes of Swedish-style massage. To see the effects of the massage on muscles, they took muscle biopsies of their legs before and after the workout and after the massage. The brief massage affected two specific genes in the muscle cells: one that decreases inflammation caused by exercise, and one that turns up production of mitochondria in the muscles. Mitochondria are the powerhouse cells that use oxygen and the broken-down products of food to generate energy needed by the cells. Now, if you don't have the money for a massage after every exercise session, grab a foam roller. They usually have them at the gym, but you can buy one for $6 to $15 online. Then roll out your muscles and effectively massage them to speed your recovery and enhance your workout results.

EAT GINGER • 1 POINT

Here's another tip to help you manage postworkout soreness. Let's say you're planning to check out that BODYSHRED class and would like to be able to sit on the toilet or raise your hands above your head the next day. Pop some ginger before getting your sweat on, and chew some afterward, too. Research indicates that 2 grams of gingerroot can effectively decrease exercise-induced muscle soreness if taken before and several days after a heavy workout. You can use fresh gingerroot or try Chimes Ginger Chews (available in many supermarkets as well as at Amazon.com).

EAT IN FRONT OF THE MIRROR • 1 POINT

One study found that when people ate in front of mirrors, the amount of food they consumed was reduced by one-third. It seems that looking yourself in the eye reflects back some of your inner goals and slimming aspirations, reminding you that you're trying to lose weight and get healthy.

FILL UP FROM THE STOVETOP •• 2 POINTS

A study out of Cornell University revealed that people eat up to 35 percent less when they fill their plate from the stovetop rather than from a serving dish placed out on the table. Hide the fine china and belly up to the burners.

DITCH THE SILVER • 1 POINT

What I mean here is, ditch your fork and switch to chopsticks. Eating with chopsticks will slow you down and can help you eat up to 25 percent fewer calories per meal. Not only will you look more cultured and worldly, you'll trim your waistline at the same time.

HAVE A COLD ONE • 1 POINT

No, not a beer—nice try. Cold water. It seems there's some truth to the age-old advice about drinking cold water to burn more calories. Apparently it's not just a diet tale. It actually does take calories to heat cold water up to body temperature. According to a recent German study, the effect is small but enough to burn an additional 17,400 calories per year, which translates into a weight loss of 5 pounds. While drinking cold water won't compensate for eating poorly, it's an easy, free way to burn a few more calories every day.

SLICE AND DICE • • 2 POINTS

Many studies have shown that when our food is cut into smaller portions, we eat less of it. By actually seeing more pieces of food on your plate, you can trick your brain into believing you're taking in more than you actually are. Research at Arizona State University found that people who were given a bagel with cream cheese that had been sliced into four pieces ate less of it than those who received a whole one.

PICTURE IT • 1 POINT

Instead of writing down every morsel you eat, after the first couple weeks of food journaling, try keeping a visual account of your daily meals. Studies suggest that snapping photos and then looking back at them can make people stop and think before indulging. Grab your cell phone and take a quick picture of what you're about to eat; pause for a second, then look at it. A simple snapshot of your heaping dish may make you think twice about having the cheesy croutons on the salad or the heaping serving of mashed potatoes. This great visual reminder may give you pause before you wreck your diet. When you get on the scale at the end of the week and you think it doesn't represent your efforts to eat less or control calories, you can go back over the photos you logged of your meals and assess where you went wrong.

SEE THE WORLD THROUGH *BLUE*-COLORED GLASSES
• 1 POINT

I mentioned in "Keep it cool" (on page 166) that colors affect our appetite. Warm colors make us hungry, while cool colors inhibit overeating. If you're out at a restaurant during the day (or night, if you don't care about looking a little odd), wear sunglasses with blue lenses. You may not feel the most attractive in blue tints, but when you're rocking your skinny jeans, you'll thank me.

WREAK HAVOC • • • 3 POINTS

This is my all-time favorite tip. It has saved me from literally thousands of unwanted calories. The minute you have any inkling that you're finished with your food, wreck it so that whatever is left over is inedible. Seriously. Pour salt all over the remains on your plate. Wad up your napkin and toss it onto your food. Do whatever you have to do to make the food impossible to eat. In fact, as I write this very tip, I just sprayed dry shampoo on the cookies Heidi brought home from her lunch and left on the kitchen table. Think about how many times you've been full but couldn't stop picking at the meal. Willpower is often a fleeting moment of bravado. The minute you have a burst of it, act immediately, as you now know it can weaken with overuse.

SLIM MYTH:

Colon flushes are great for weight loss and detoxing.

FAST FACT: No true medical research supports any health benefit whatsoever from colonics. The only weight loss a colonic promotes will be the removal of waste from your bowel. Ironically, in the long run this procedure can actually inhibit the action of your body's *true* weight-loss helper: probiotic balance. A colonic can deprive your microflora (good gut bacteria) of vital nutrition, and gut bacteria play a role in weight management and a healthy digestive system. My last thought on colonics: they have also been shown to create electrolyte imbalances, which can result in nausea, vomiting, bloating, muscle cramps, and, in extremely severe cases, seizures. Please avoid this kooky trend at all costs. Who wants someone sticking a hose in their bum anyway? I mean, seriously.

Now, if you're one of those people who hates wasting food, especially when you're eating out (I have this issue too), gain some perspective. The food you don't eat will not be shipped to starving people across the ocean; but if you eat it, it's going to your gut, thighs, or butt. You choose.

T2 •• 2 POINTS

In "Engage in teatime" (page 171), we talked about teas that help curb cravings and hunger. But the following powerhouse teas actually help burn fat and up your fat metabolism! Try them:

- *King Peony White Tea.* The active ingredient in this tea is EGCG, which inhibits fat storage and promotes lipolysis. Drink 2 cups after a heavy meal. Plus theanine, an amino acid found in white and green tea leaves, can increase energy and help reduce anxiety and stress.
- *Loose Leaf Pu'erh.* Pu'erh tea, known as the "drinkable antique," comes from the mountains of Yunnan, in southern China, where the ancient tea trees grow. Pu'erh is different from

other teas because, like wine, its taste improves with age, becoming more flavorful and mellow. Scientists claim that there's an activating enzyme in this tea that will literally shrink fat cells. Drink 1 or 2 cups in the morning for optimal results.

PUT A BOW ON IT •• 2 POINTS

This is a little trick I learned from a French friend, and it works great. When you go out to dinner, tie a ribbon around your waist, under your clothes. As you become full, you'll feel the ribbon tighten. This will create an awareness of your body and remind you to pay conscious attention to how much you're consuming. It will keep you from needlessly and heedlessly overindulging.

EAT PUNGENT FOOD, AND NATURALLY TAKE FEWER BITES • 1 POINT

We already discussed (in "Spice it up," page 88) that you should be using herbs and spices to flavor your food because they're healthy for you as well as extremely low-calorie alternatives to sauces, sugars, and salt. But their benefits don't stop there. A report in the journal *Flavour* showed that strong food aromas can help you eat 5 to 10 percent less of your meal. Apparently, strong food smells make people unconsciously take smaller bites, to regulate the amount of flavor they experience. Try the following suggestions out, and see how they work for you:

- Add ⅔ teaspoon of rosemary to a steak, chicken, or salmon fillet.
- Add ¼ cup diced apples, 1 teaspoon grated ginger, and ½ teaspoon cinnamon to oatmeal or pancakes.
- Marinate a chicken breast in plain Greek yogurt with 1 tablespoon freshly chopped mint.
- Stir ¼ teaspoon Chinese five-spice powder into a cup of bean, turkey, or grass-fed beef chili.

- Crush a couple cloves of garlic and add them to your pasta sauce.

DON'T HIDE THE EVIDENCE •• 2 POINTS

Leave snack wrappers and containers on your desk to remind you of how much you've been eating. I find this keeps me from grazing and mindless munching because I realize there's no possible way I'm actually hungry.

DAINTY PLATES, PLEASE •• 2 POINTS

No plate you eat off of should be platter-sized. Your dinner plate should be no bigger than 10 inches across. A study from Cornell University found that people who ate off smaller plates believed that they were eating an average of 18 percent more calories than they actually were. Those eating off bigger dinner plates didn't have the same portion distortion. You really do eat with your eyes, not your stomach. So hit Ikea and scoop up some smaller plates—stat!

NO CARBS AT NIGHT ••• 3 POINTS

I know I always tell you to eat balanced portions of healthy proteins, fats, and carbs throughout your day, but there actually is *one* exception. I want you to cut all carbs (except greens) at least three hours before bed. In fact, if you can cut them out of dinner altogether, that would be even better. The reason is that you release most of your body's fat-burning, anti-aging, muscle-building hormone, human growth hormone (HGH) during your first cycle of sleep. Starchy and sugary carbs release more insulin, and insulin drives down HGH levels. So carbs before bed can actually rob you of precious HGH production.

AVOID KITSCHY-SOUNDING FOOD •• 2 POINTS

This is particularly applicable during holidays. Every time there's a frickin' holiday, the big food companies and fast-food restaurant

SLIM MYTH:

Don't eat before bed.

FAST FACT: While many diets tell you not to eat after a certain time in the evening, that couldn't be more irrelevant with regard to your diet. Calories don't tell time. Researchers have often studied when people consumed their last meal in conjunction with their bedtime and found zero indication that it made any impact whatsoever on their weight.

In a study at the Dunn Clinical Nutrition Centre in Cambridge, U.K., volunteers were placed in a whole-body calorimeter, which measures calories burned and stored. They were fed a large lunch and a small evening meal for one test period, then a small lunch and a large evening meal during a second test period. The results revealed the large meal eaten late at night did not make the body store more fat.

The only reason late-night eating is associated with obesity is that you're usually *overeating* by the time you eat that late. You've had your three main meals and a snack, and now you're going back for more. It's the amount of food that's making you fat, not the fact that it's just before bed.

chains roll out ridiculously titled meals with obscene calorie counts. At Christmas time, IHOP offers its Eggnog Pancakes, which contain 2,150 calories for a plate of four (nearly double the calories of their regular pancake stack). How about the holiday-themed Reese's Peanut Butter Snowman, a bar that weighs in at 760 calories (3.5 times the amount of a regular Reese's two-pack)? Then at Thanksgiving Dunkin' Donuts offers the Warm Cinnamon Swirl Muffin, which contains 630 calories and a third more sugar than the chain's average muffin. This kind of celebratory supersizing happens for every holiday, from the Valentine's Day heart-shaped Heartbreaker Pizza at Papa Murphy's, to the Fourth of July Declaration Burger at the FUKU Burger chain. And all of them have more sugar, calories, and crap than the regular everyday versions. Do yourself and your ass a favor, and find another way to celebrate.

BE ADAPTABLE •• 2 POINTS

Give your taste buds time to adapt to healthier foods. When I intro-
duce *Biggest Loser* contestants to my favorite foods as part of their
regular meal plan, they often make gag-faces or stare at me incred-
ulously. Their taste buds
have to adapt to the new
food and detox from all the
fattening junk food that
has addicted them to crap.

> **EZ CALORIE CUT**
>
> Love a hamburger with the works? Eat half the bun, eat the whole burger, and skimp on the condiments and cheese. **CUT: 150 CALORIES**

These foods have the same type of pull as cigarettes. To a smoker,
cigarettes are heaven; to a nonsmoker, they taste like a cotton ball
dragged through the gutter. A nonsmoker smokes one cigarette
and is left with a headache and nausea. Same when it comes to
addictive foods—getting off them can be hard. But once you're off,
they taste gross to you—too sweet or too salty—and reintroducing
them can make you feel sick.

If the switch from ultra-fattening foods to ultra-slimming foods
is too much of a jolt to your system and psyche, try to baby-step
your way through it. Here are two examples of what I mean:

1. First switch from fried chicken to barbecue chicken. (You've cut
most of the fat calories but still have some sugar and salt in the
sauce.) Then graduate to chicken parmesan, with no more than 4
teaspoons of cheese. (Now you've eliminated the sugar.) Last, try
herb-crusted, baked, or grilled chicken. You've now added all the
health benefits of the herbs, and you've cut out the sugar, the salt,
and about 300 calories since that fried chicken.

2. Go from an iceberg wedge salad covered in blue cheese or
ranch dressing and croutons to a romaine salad with one tablespoon of creamy dressing and no croutons. Romaine has far more
metabolism-boosting nutrients, and you'll cut at least 100 calories

by decreasing the dressing amount. Then switch over to spinach salad with balsamic vinaigrette on the side. Now you're getting heart-healthy fat from the olive oil, and by putting the dressing on the side, you'll save at least another 100 calories.

BETTER TOGETHER: COMBINING FOODS FOR MAXIMUM FAT BURN •• 2 POINTS

Want to get the most out of your food? Well, this is the right section to come to, as it's all about how to combine certain foods together to amp up your fat-burning potential. I don't want you to confuse this concept with the ideas from that 1980s book *Fit for Life,* which espoused a bunch of nonsense about not consuming starches and proteins together because they require different digestive environments (acid vs. alkaline). According to believers, eating these foods at the same time stresses the digestive system, causing the carbs (starches) to ferment and the proteins to basically rot. Utter bull. However, there are certain key foods that, when combined together, offer optimal nutrient absorption, ultimately helping you to burn more fat. Here are the five key food combos for better fat utilization:

- **Spinach and citrus.** Vitamin C (found in citrus) helps the body absorb nonheme, or plant-based, iron (found in spinach). This is really important for women (as our monthly visitor can occasionally make us borderline anemic) and for vegetarians. Steam up some spinach, then sauté it very quickly with a tiny bit of olive oil and lemon juice. Or throw some mandarin orange slices in with your next spinach salad. Iron is vital to maintaining exercise stamina, as it plays a critical role in oxygen transport and fuel utilization. Remember, the harder you train, the more calories you'll burn.
- **Vegetables and healthy fat.** Prepare vegetables with a tiny bit of healthy fat, like olive oil, for maximum absorption of pro-

tective phytochemicals. Many nutrients are fat-soluble and therefore are better absorbed by the body when consumed with healthy fats. Hormones are predominantly synthesized from the building blocks of vitamins and minerals, so better absorption will support everything from proper thyroid function to estrogen and testosterone balance. All three play a major role in how your body burns and stores fat.

- **Vitamin D and calcium.** Vitamin D helps the body absorb calcium, so be sure to buy dairy products fortified with it. Many brands of coconut milk also have vitamin D added to them. If the process of fortification worries you, you can eat a calcium-rich food, then catch a bit of sun. Current research points to vitamin D as crucial for heart health and as a potential defense against hypertension, cancer, and several autoimmune diseases. Research also suggests that diets rich in calcium can help reduce body fat. Instead of going crazy pounding glasses of milk and cubes of cheese, utilize this trick to optimize your calcium intake without adding the extra calories.

- **Red wine or grapes, and fish or nuts.** A few ounces of red wine or a handful of grapes can enhance the absorption of the omega-3 fats in fish and nuts. Omega-3 has long been lauded for benefiting heart health and brainpower, and now we know it plays a role in weight loss. Fish oil contains docosahexaenoic acid (DHA) and eicosapentaenoic (EPA) fatty acids. Researchers in Australia report that those who take omega-3 fish oil and exercise moderately burn more fat and lose more weight than those who exercise but don't take the fish oil. The theory is that fish oil improves blood flow to muscles, which increases the benefits of exercise. In that study, those who took the fish oil exercised for 45 minutes three times a week. In addition, EFAs (essential fatty acids) produce hormones called eicosanoids that regulate digestion and insulin production. Insulin promotes fat storage. When people regularly consume omega-3 fish oil, insulin levels drop 50 percent lower, allowing individuals to use a higher percentage of fat for energy. (More on fish oil in a few moments.)

- **Protein and starchy or sugary carbs.** When you consume food, it goes through a complex process of digestion and absorption. The body breaks down high-glycemic-index carbs (sugar and starch) quickly, causing blood sugar to spike. As blood sugar levels rise, insulin enters the bloodstream to deliver sugar molecules to their appropriate cell destinations. The problem is that when the cells don't use the sugar immediately for fuel, they store it as fat. So stabilizing insulin and blood sugar levels is another key to weight management. When carbohydrates are consumed along with protein, the digestive process slows down. The carbohydrate sugars take a longer time to be absorbed into the bloodstream, leveling the rise in blood sugar rather than giving you a sugar spike, thus helping to control hunger and decrease the promotion of fat storage. So if you're having oatmeal for breakfast, throw in a couple of scrambled egg whites on the side. If you're eating baked chips and salsa as a snack, roll up a couple of turkey slices to have with them.

Slim Trickery

While it's become unpopular to suggest that certain supplements aid in weight loss, the reality is, some do. Let's distinguish right off the difference between pharmaceuticals and supplements. A supplement is a naturally occurring thing within our foods, like caffeine, omega-3s, chromium picolinate, or quercetin. A pharmaceutical, on the other hand, may have originated from a plant or animal but has been isolated and synthesized to the point of being unrecognizable, subsequently becoming a new chemical that can be patented.

I never want you to take pharmaceutical drugs like Phentermine, Alli, or Qysimia for two reasons. First, taking these pills is no way to approach lasting weight loss. You need to learn how to eat well and move more efficiently to attain and maintain your slim. Second, they're dangerous and have scary side effects: headaches, back pain, abdominal pain, palpitations, constipation, nausea, thirst, joint problems, insomnia, dizziness, anxiety, depression, rash, acne, primary pulmonary hypertension, regurgitant cardiac valvular disease, elevated blood pressure, restlessness, diarrhea, impotence—and so on. Not cool. These drugs should be avoided whenever possible.

But if you're eating a healthy, sound diet, working out hard, and just want a little extra edge, research suggests there are safe and natural ways to get it. That's what the following is about: supplementing safely to boost your metabolic function and exercise endurance.

CHEAT YOUR WAY SLIM

GET BUZZED—DRINK CAFFEINE • • • 3 POINTS

I have to give you this one with the caveat of talking to your doctor before imbibing. Anyone who experiences anxiety or has high blood pressure or any other health-related condition that's negatively affected by caffeine shouldn't drink beverages with it. That aside, if you don't suffer from any such issue, caffeine, when taken in the right form and the right dosage, has a ton of health benefits, from helping to fight pancreatic cancer and type 2 diabetes to fending off

Alzheimer's, Parkinson's, and dementia. A number of studies have shown that drinking coffee daily may even contribute to longevity! Remember: coffee is "calorie free," until you start adding the chocolate, cream, mocha, and sugar.

But with regard to our slim agenda, the most important benefit of caffeine is that it helps us burn fat. According to the Mayo Clinic, it provides short-term appetite suppression and stimulates the nervous system, resulting in a mild calorie burn. But this calorie use isn't where its true fat-burning potential lies. For caffeine to be most effective in the slimming department, you have to combine it with exercise. It dramatically enhances fitness performance because it lowers our perception of the intensity or difficulty of our efforts. Thus we are able to exercise at a higher intensity for longer, without actually feeling like we are working harder. And of course, the harder we work in the gym, the more calories we can burn during the workout and even hours after it's over—particularly when we are resistance training. Plus, caffeine spares muscle glycogen (stored carbohydrates) and promotes the use of fat stores as energy.

The key to constructive caffeine consumption is to consume no more than 400 milligrams a day, preferably divided in 2 separate "doses" of 200 milligrams a pop. (In total, that's equivalent to two strong cups of coffee.) Have one when you first wake up, then another, roughly 45 minutes before you exercise, unless it's past three p.m. (Disregard this if you're one of those rare individuals who can drink coffee regardless of the time of day and still sleep at night—notice I used the word *rare*.) Be sure not to consume more than 400 milligrams because too much caffeine can have the opposite of our desired effect. It can tax adrenal glands, stress us out, release the belly fat hormone cortisol, and disrupt sleep patterns. Bad, bad, bad.

Coffee is an okay source of caffeine, but not ideal. Coffee can raise "bad" cholesterol levels and dehydrate you, and if it's not organic, it can have high levels of pesticides. I suggest a natural caffeine supplement like EBoost. I fell in love with this product so much, I actually invested in the company. Here's why: it contains around 160 milligrams of caffeine from green tea, but produces none of the harmful side effects of coffee. Plus, it has electrolytes to help fend off dehydration as well as antioxidants and immunity boosters for overall health. You get lots of bang for your buck.

GET YOUR "MOO" ON •• 2 POINTS

Recent research suggests that 3 or 4 daily servings of low-fat dairy products can boost your body's fat-burning potential. Numerous studies have shown that organic dairy-rich diets (based on milk protein, aka whey) may help weight loss, improving the body's ability to burn fat, and it may do so better than calcium supplementation. But two studies from the University of Tennessee, published in 2011, suggest that eating calcium-rich products causes a rise in body heat, causing fat to burn more easily. In another analysis, researchers found that dieting women who received 1,000 milligrams of calcium supplements each day lost, on average, more weight and more body fat than women taking a placebo. Although the differences in the amount of weight and fat lost by the two groups were not huge, the data suggests a correlation between calcium intake and fat metabolism. Researchers say this is because

SLIM MYTH:
Chocolate milk is a great workout recovery drink.

FAST FACT: Chocolate milk makes you fat and has hardly any nutritional benefits. It's loaded with sugar, hormones, and antibiotics. Even if you get it organic, it still has tons of sugar and calories. A study supports the claim that chocolate milk has "just the right amount of protein and carbs" to fuel your recovery. Absurd. Guess who funded that study? The National Dairy Council and the National Fluid Milk Processor Promotion Board. So I question its validity. Again, when something sounds too good to be true—it's BS. There are much healthier, cleaner sources of both protein and carbs with less sugar and calories. Try a whey protein shake instead, with some fresh fruit.

calcium stored in fat cells plays an important role in fat storage and breakdown.

If you're using calcium supplements, it's important to choose those with added vitamin D, zinc, and magnesium, which help the body to better absorb the calcium. If you want to get your calcium from food, here are a few calcium-rich ones to choose from: organic low-fat Greek yogurt, organic cheese, organic milk, and dark leafy greens (especially for the vegans in the house).

CATCH SOME RAYS •• 2 POINTS

Vitamin D is the latest fat-burning-supplement breakthrough with real scientific credibility. A ton of research published to date suggests that vitamin D deficiency contributes to obesity and, conversely, that getting adequate vitamin D helps fend it off. When you have enough vitamin D in your bloodstream, fat cells slow their efforts to make and store fat. But when vitamin D levels are low, levels of parathyroid hormone (PTH) and calcitrol rise, and high levels of these two hormones throw your body into fat-storage mode. In fact, a Norwegian study found that elevated PTH levels increased a man's risk of becoming overweight by 40 percent.

Vitamin D has also been shown to work with calcium to reduce the production of cortisol, that pesky stress hormone that causes you to store belly fat. When you have adequate vitamin D levels, your body releases more leptin, the hormone that conveys a "We're full, stop eating" message to your brain. An Australian study showed that people who ate a breakfast high in D and calcium blunted their appetites for the next 24 hours. Last, vitamin D deficiency is linked to insulin resistance, which leads to hunger and overeating.

The sun is our absolute best source of vitamin D, so your number-one option is to spend 15 minutes a day in the sun during off-peak hours (later afternoon). If this is not an option for you, then take a supplement, one that contains not only vitamin D but calcium and magnesium. It's very easy to find a supplement that combines these nutrients. One thousand international units (IUs) of vitamin D is the suggested amount to consume each day. The brand I take is called Bone Strength by New Chapter Organics. It has 1,000 IUs of vitamin D_3 with calcium and magnesium.

Another way to pump up your vitamin D and calcium intake without supplements is to eat yogurt, and I mean healthy yogurt, free of HFCS, high sugar, and additives. Personally I love the consistency of Oikos Greek yogurt. Researchers at the University of Tennessee have found that dieters who ate three servings of yogurt a day lost 22 percent more weight and 61 percent more body fat than those in the study who only cut calories and didn't include calcium supplementation. Safe to say, yogurt is a solid source of both vitamin D and calcium, helps burn fat, and promotes weight loss. There are countless ways to include it in your diet, too, if you don't enjoy eating a container of it. Substitute yogurt for mayonnaise when you're making salad dressing. Use it in a smoothie. Mix it in with whole-grain cereal for breakfast instead of using milk.

ENGAGE IN FISHY BUSINESS •• 2 POINTS

Fish oil offers a wide array of health benefits, and you should be supplementing with it, if you're not allergic. Recent research suggests that fish oil may help you lose fat and build muscle. Several animal studies have shown clearly that diets rich in omega-3 fatty acids, specifically eicosapentaenoic acid (EPA) and docosahexaenoic acid (DHA), found largely in the oil from cold-water fish, lead to significantly lower total body fat stores than those of diets rich in other fatty acids. The exact reasons are unknown, but these studies show that EPA and DHA suppress "lipogenic gene expression" and increase mitochondrial lipid oxidization. (Sorry, I know I promised no science lessons.) Basically this means that omega-3s suppress your body's fat-storing tendencies and support and enhance its fat-burning ability. There's limited evidence that consistent fish oil supplementation in your diet can also reduce cortisol levels; if that turns out to be true, then decreasing cortisol levels could potentially reduce body fat percentage.

If you don't regularly eat fish (especially deep-water fatty fish), or if you eat too many processed foods and oils (even though I told you not to), seriously consider adding a fish oil supplement to your daily regimen. Top brands like Barlean's, Nature's Made, Nordic Naturals, Solgar, and NOW brands all have strict policies and procedures regarding the manufacture of fish oil, which undergoes molecular distillation to remove mercury and other harmful contaminants. Seeing a decrease in fat and an increase in muscle requires taking 2 to 3 grams of total EPA and DHA per day. And don't forget, combining a few ounces of red wine or a handful of grapes with your omega-3's enhances your body's absorption. One caveat: anyone taking a blood thinner should speak with their doctor and discuss whether it's safe to take this supplement and if so at what dose.

TAKE YOUR "TWO-A-DAY" •• 2 POINTS

How can a multi affect your weight? We know that hormones and healthy biochemistry are built through healthy nutrition. Thyroid hormones, for example, which affect your metabolism and weight, require selenium, zinc, and iodine in adequate quantities. Although in a perfect world we would get our nutrition by eating healthy food, often our diets aren't varied enough or organic enough to get the nutrients we need for optimal functionality. For this reason, a quality multivitamin is a great idea, not just for your health but also for your physique. The key is quality! Cheap vitamins are not only useless, they can be downright bad for you if they're loaded with artificial crap like trans fats, sweeteners, and artificial colors. If you're going to use this tip, spend money on a quality supplement, and make sure to check the ingredients to make sure it's crap free.

Rainbow, New Chapter Organics, Source Naturals, and Ultimate Nutrition are all good brands.

FEED YOUR GUT •• 2 POINTS

The little bugs in your gut are super for your overall health, but they also make great weight-loss buddies. Probiotics boost your body's ability to absorb vitamins and minerals, and they change the health and balance of your gut bacteria, subsequently aiding in weight loss. This absorption benefit is incredibly important, because as I've mentioned, vitamins and minerals are key for synthesizing hormones. To make thyroid hormone, for example (a massive metabolic regulator), you need iodine, zinc, and selenium. If your body can't properly absorb these minerals, your thyroid function will suffer.

With regard to the exact role that healthy gut bacteria play in promoting weight loss, researchers aren't sure what the mechanism is, but the proof is in the findings. In 2006, Stanford University researchers found that obese people had different gut bacteria ratios than those who maintained a healthy weight, a solid indication that gut flora play a role in overall weight. Another study carried out by researchers at Lund University in Sweden found that adding probiotic bacteria to the diet reduced weight gain. And yet another study suggested that probiotics may help regulate the process by which energy is used by the body. One more: the Center for Health Policy at the Stanford University School of Medicine found that the use of probiotics can help gastric-bypass patients lose weight more quickly. Makes sense to beef up on these beneficial bacteria, doesn't it?

FIBER UP •• 2 POINTS

If you want to squelch hunger, eat fiber; or if you're still adjusting your new diet to include high-fiber foods, take a fiber supplement. A recent study found that overweight and obese people who took

FAST FACT: I love when people who have absolutely no knowledge of nutrition or weight loss say this stuff to me. It's utterly illogical. The inability to "process" foods would mean the foods are not metabolized and calories would not be absorbed. This would lead to weight loss, not gain. By the way, even if you have a food allergy, no scientific evidence suggests that food allergy causes weight gain. Discomfort, yes. Bloating, maybe. Weight gain, no.

a fiber supplement each day reported less hunger after meals than people taking a placebo. This is because fiber helps to "delay gastric emptying," which means food stays in the stomach longer, making you feel fuller for an extended period of time.

Ideally, you would eat more vegetables to up your fiber intake, but if you decide instead to increase your fiber with supplements, be sure to do it slowly (don't go overboard), and drink plenty of fluids to avoid becoming constipated. The National Academy of Sciences' Institute of Medicine recommends that men under the age of 50 consume 38 grams of fiber a day, and 30 grams a day over age 50. Women under 50 should consume at least 25 grams of fiber per day, and 21 grams per day over age 50. Most people get only about half of this amount. You can get fancy with your fiber supplements, but a simple bottle of psyllium husk capsules will do the trick nicely. Take as the bottle directs.

BEAT THE BLOAT • 1 POINT

Bloating makes you feel very uncomfortable. Even if you're thin, living through that time of the month, eating a high-sodium meal, or being low in potassium can make anyone feel chubby. The solution: drink water. The more water you drink, the less water you hold. Also, reduce your sodium intake to 1,500 milligrams a day, and eat potassium-rich foods. Doing so will help to flush out your body, as well as eliminate any bloating caused by too much sodium. You can instantly feel and look slimmer just from this simple change of habit.

Here are some great bloat-busting food options that are

potassium-rich: coconut water, banana, papaya, yogurt, lima beans, cantaloupe, and beets. If you don't have the calories to spare, you can also just take a supplement like Electro Mix (available at any health food store), which has 400 milligrams of potassium with none of the calories.

FUEL YOUR FIT • 1 POINT

I've talked at great length and in detail in my books and on my website about the important role nutrients play in metabolic function, immunity, and overall wellness. Now I want to specifically address which foods (and the nutrients in them) support and enhance fitness performance. Remember, the harder you train, the more calories you're going to burn.

- **Iron.** Iron increases blood count by aiding in the formation of red blood cells, which transport oxygen throughout our bodies, thus improving our total oxygen capacity and facilitating a more intense workout.

  Found in grass-fed beef, egg yolks, dark leafy greens.

- **Quercetin.** According to recent studies, quercetin provides a moderate improvement in performance/endurance in trained athletes and a more significant effect in untrained individuals. This is thought to happen because quercetin boosts mitochondrial biogenesis, which in turn boosts VO_2max (the maximum amount of oxygen an individual can utilize), thereby enhancing endurance exercise capacity. Researchers think seasoned athletes don't see much of a bump in performance because they've already maxed out their mitochondrial production. Bottom line, you could supplement with quercetin in pill form, but eating foods that have it certainly can't hurt either, especially if you're just starting out on your exercise regimen.

  Found in apple skins and berries.

- **Nitric oxide.** Nitric oxide reduces the amount of oxygen burned by the body during a workout, subsequently boosting the body's power and endurance. One source is beetroot juice, which researchers believe may work to boost stamina by affecting how the body processes nitrate into nitric oxide. Another source is peppers and spicy foods that contain capsaicin; it activates a receptor found in the lining of blood vessels that leads to an increase in the production of nitric oxide.

  Found in beets, jalapeños, and cayenne peppers.

- **CoQ10 and CoQH.** Coenzyme Q10 (CoQ10) and coenzyme QH (a more stabilized form of CoQ10) are found only in trace amounts in foods, particularly meats and fish. They exist, however, in all the cells in your body. CoQ10 and CoQH influence the mitochondria in your body's cells, which are responsible for converting fatty acids and glucose into energy. Specifically, they're vital to making adenosine triphosphate (ATP), the energy source for your body (which gives you the power and stamina to hit your workout hard). And as I've said: the harder you work, the more calories you burn!

  Found in grass-fed beef, pork, chicken, salmon, sardines, and mackerel.

....

Fashion Statements

DRESS SLIM

Let me be crystal clear about this next piece of advice: there's no article of clothing or fashion strategy that will literally take weight off your body (which is why I'm not giving points for the tips in this section). The clothes you wear, however, and the way you wear them can make you look 10 pounds lighter in seconds. I'm the farthest thing from a fashionista, but the following secrets were given to me by top stylists in L.A., Miami, and New York—and they work! When I learned this stuff and saw the immediate difference it made in the way my body looked, I thought, *Why isn't this information common knowledge?*

While it's crucial that you do the actual "heavy lifting" when it comes to achieving your sexy slim physique, a little optical illusion here and there is a great way to enhance the results of your slim lifestyle. I'm slim, and I use these tips *all* the time. So pay attention, and then play dress-up.

WEAR A V-NECK
It lengthens your neck and shows off your collarbone.

GO MONOCHROMATIC
Dressing in one color head to toe is the easiest slim trick of all because it creates one long, clean line and doesn't break your body up into separate visual parts. It also makes you look taller. This tip is a great one for us petite people.

BUY ONLY WHAT YOU CAN MOVE IN
Don't stuff yourself into clothes that don't fit. If you do, it will cause rolls and bulges even on the slimmest of women. If you have to wiggle around in the dressing room to get it on, put it back on the rack.

PRACTICE THE ART OF CAMOUFLAGE
Darker colors will minimize and lighter or shiny ones will highlight. So if you have a thicker waist, wear a brown or black belt. If you want to play down a large double-D chest, avoid wearing a gold or silver blouse.

CHOOSE FLATTERING FABRICS

When you're trying to deemphasize a "problem area," wear a crisp fabric, not clingy materials that show everything you're trying to disguise. Conversely, when you want to show off an area of your body that you feel good about, wear the clingy materials. If you have killer legs but a little muffin top, opt for fitted jeans with a crisp tucked-in shirt as opposed to the stretchy wool sweater and baggy jeans.

DON'T GO BAGGY

Big shapes make you look bigger. I'm telling you, this is true. I learned this one firsthand on a bikini shoot for *Shape* magazine. I wanted to wear the cute boy-short bathing suit, and they wanted me in a small bikini. I insisted that bigger was better, but when I saw the pictures, I realized I was wrong. The bigger the suit, the bigger I looked. The directive you should follow here comes straight from famed costume designer Edith Head: "Wear clothes loose enough to prove you're a lady, but tight enough to prove you're a woman."

TAILOR YOUR CLOTHES

You can't expect every size 8 to fit every size 8 woman. Get a tailor you love and trust to fit your nicer clothes to your body. I know this can get pricey, but once you have a few beautifully tailored staples in your wardrobe, you'll be prepared for any event and fashion necessity.

GO SMALL WITH PRINTS

This one came from a *Redbook* cover shoot I did, when the stylist put me in jeans with a paisley pattern on them. I was extremely resistant, thinking these jeans were going to make me look like I had thick legs. Wrong. They looked great and slimming, and here's why: the smaller the pattern, the smaller you look. Thin stripes, tiny polka dots, little paisleys are the way to go when wearing a print.

BELT IT

Every single stylist has told me to draw attention to my waist. This is because it accentuates the smallest part of a woman. Tossing a belt on or over just about anything will help give your body a slimmer profile—just don't overcinch. That's how muffin tops are born.

PICK THE RIGHT POCKETS

The ideal size for a super-sexy bum pocket is no smaller than your palm and no bigger than your hand. Stray outside these guidelines, and you're playing with fire (the illusion of a much bigger booty and not in a good way). And make sure that the bottom of your pocket never dips lower than your actual bum.

GO SAME ON SAME

Pair any color pant with the same color shoe for longer-looking legs. This also works with nude shoes if you're wearing a dress.

INVEST IN THE PERFECT PUSH-UP

This one has been a life changer for me. I can't tell you how many rumors on the Internet started circling that I got a boob job after I found the right bra. Higher, bigger boobs in seconds with no surgery at minimal cost—I'll take it. Plus, the higher your boobs sit, the slimmer your waist looks. Don't take this upon yourself. Get professional help. Go to an expert, and get yourself professionally measured. They do this at any major department store in the lingerie section or at specific lingerie stores like Victoria's Secret. Although you might be slightly embarrassed in the moment, it's so worth it.

ADD IT UP, DROP IT OFF

GIVE YOURSELF 3 POINTS

☐ Don't be a party animal.

☐ Make a date with your scale.

☐ Limit TV time.

☐ Wreak havoc.

☐ No carbs at night.

☐ Get buzzed—drink caffeine.

GIVE YOURSELF 2 POINTS

☐ Standing room only.

☐ Fidget.

☐ Get it together.

☐ Tread wisely.

☐ Fill up from the stovetop.

☐ Slice and dice.

☐ T2.

☐ Put a bow on it.

☐ Don't hide the evidence.

☐ Dainty plates, please.

☐ Avoid kitschy-sounding food.

☐ Be adaptable.

☐ Better together: combining foods for maximum fat burn.

☐ Get your "moo" on.

☐ Catch some rays.

☐ Engage in fishy business.

☐ Take your "two-a-day."

☐ Feed your gut.

☐ Fiber up.

GIVE YOURSELF 1 POINT

☐ Be hot and cold.

☐ Kick-start your week on the weekend.

☐ Be minty fresh.

☐ Cold hands, killer workout.

☐ Be a rock 'n' roller.

☐ Eat ginger.

☐ Eat in front of the mirror.

☐ Ditch the silver.

☐ Have a cold one.

☐ Picture it.

☐ See the world through *blue-*colored glasses.

☐ Eat pungent food, and naturally take fewer bites.

☐ Beat the bloat.

☐ Fuel your fit.

_____ **Total *points* for Chapter 7**

_____ **Total number of *tips* I'm incorporating**

CHAPTER 8

THE FINAL COUNTDOWN

Here we are. You made it to the end. Congrats! Now, before we both break our arms patting you on the back, let's see where you fall in the grand slim scheme. Knowing how much you've achieved, and how geared you are to continued success, will help keep you headed in the right direction as you settle into this new way of life.

We're going to evaluate your slim life in two ways. First, we're going to look at your total point score, based on adding up the numeric value of the tips you chose to follow in each chapter. Then we'll figure the percentage of total tips in this book that you're choosing to utilize.

Why bother to do this? Assigning points to your habits does a couple of positive, concrete things. It helps you see which strategies are more powerful than others. It allows you to see the results of the choices you make or don't make, and it gives me the ability to help you fine-tune your plan so that you're 100 percent set up for success.

One of the key ways we can fine-tune your success is by analyzing your tip percentage (the number of tips in *Slim for Life* that you have chosen to follow). By taking into account both your accumulative, total tip score and your tip percentage, we can get a rock-solid idea of not only the quantity but the quality of the tips you've selected. For example, if your points total in the 200-to-300 range but you have a low tip percentage, it shows me you have chosen more of the power tips, the tips with a value of 3, than 1s. Conversely, if you have a lower overall score but a higher tip percentage, it shows me you haven't really committed to the power tips. These ideas are the most potent and multitasking slim changers in the book. Before I say more on that, let's address how often you should be employing the tips you've picked.

At the very beginning of the book, I told you that you didn't need to choose all the tips, or do the ones you chose all the time. Before we get down to the nitty-gritty and see how your choices literally add up, let me clarify how often you should be engaging in the new behaviors you've chosen to adopt. Remember the 80/20 rule? I'd love to see you following the suggestions you've chosen 80 percent of the time. This is really the magic formula that allows room for fun and pleasure without jeopardizing your results.

You ready to see your score? Me too! Let's get calculating.

POINT SCORE TOTAL

Grab a pen and paper, or your laptop, and go back to the end of each chapter. We are going to add up your total point score from all the chapters combined. Remember, each tip was assigned a point value of 3, 2, or 1. The number of total points available in each chapter is the sum of these point values. List your results here.

CHAPTER 1   Total Points Available = 57:   **Your Point Score** _____

CHAPTER 2   Total Points Available = 52:   **Your Point Score** _____

CHAPTER 3   Total Points Available = 113:   **Your Point Score** _____

CHAPTER 4   Total Points Available = 116:   **Your Point Score** _____

CHAPTER 5   Total Points Available = 77:   **Your Point Score** _____

CHAPTER 6   Total Points Available = 118:   **Your Point Score** _____

CHAPTER 7   Total Points Available = 70:   **Your Point Score** _____

Wait, before we count up your absolute total point score, guess what? I have some bonus points to give you. I was always big on extra credit as a kid. I didn't assign point values for the tips on Budget and Dressing Slim, or in the EZ Calorie Cuts and NEAT sidebars, but if you're employing them, that should count for a little something. Actions like joining a food co-op, comparison shopping or dressing in ways that flatter your physique don't themselves burn fat, but they do show that you're being proactive and choosing to focus on yourself and your overall wellness—and that's a big deal in the scheme of things.

If you sincerely plan on incorporating at least half the suggestions in the NEAT sidebars and the EZ Calorie Cuts, along with several recommendations from both the money-saving and dressing-slim sections, then give yourself 10 bonus points. If you're going to do half of what I just suggested, take 5. Less than that, you're out of luck—no extra credit for you. Don't get me wrong, I still want you to do these things as often as possible. Even a handful will make a difference, but for them to have a significant impact, you'll need to engage in more of them. Since they aren't tips that directly affect your slim, their true potency is in their collective power.

Okay, now let's add all this up!

ALL CHAPTERS   Total Points Available: 603

Bonus Points Available: 10

(ADD UP THE 7 TOTALS YOU LISTED ABOVE AND POST BELOW)

Your Total Point Score _____

TOTAL TIPS CHECKED

Before I explain what your total point score means, we need to figure out what *percentage of tips* you'll be utilizing out of all that are
applicable and have point values. There are 289 tips for which you
can receive point values. I've created a chart below so you can list
the number of tips you're using from each chapter. Go back once
more to your scorecard from each chapter and add up the number of "valued" tips you selected, and list that number below here.
Wondering what I'm up to now?

Although this doesn't affect your point score, what it tells me
in conjunction with your total point score is what *types* of choices
you've made in terms of the ideas you plan on utilizing. This will,
again, enable me to provide more accurate feedback and amplify
your results—should you require it.

CHAPTER 1	Total Tips = 28:	**Tips checked =** _____
CHAPTER 2	Total Tips = 25:	**Tips checked =** _____
CHAPTER 3	Total Tips = 49:	**Tips checked =** _____
CHAPTER 4	Total Tips = 54:	**Tips checked =** _____
CHAPTER 5	Total Tips = 37:	**Tips checked =** _____
CHAPTER 6	Total Tips = 56:	**Tips checked =** _____
CHAPTER 7	Total Tips = 39:	**Tips checked =** _____
	TOTAL TIPS = 288	**Total Tips checked =** _____

Let's take a look at what this means by figuring out what tip percentage you've chosen to engage; then I'll explain what this means
in regard to your big picture.

- If you checked off between 1 and 29 total tips, you've chosen to do between 1 and 10 percent of the suggestions in this book.

- If you checked off between 30 and 58 tips, you've chosen to do between 10 and 20 percent of the suggestions in this book.

- If you checked off between 59 and 87 tips, you've chosen to do between 21 and 30 percent of the suggestions in this book.

- If you checked off between 88 and 116 tips, you've chosen to do between 31 and 40 percent of the suggestions in this book.

- If you checked off between 117 and 145 tips, you've chosen to do between 41 and 50 percent of the suggestions in this book.

- If you checked off between 146 and 174 tips, you've chosen to do between 51 and 60 percent of the suggestions in this book.

- If you checked off between 175 and 203 tips, you've chosen to do between 61 and 70 percent of the suggestions in this book.

- If you checked off between 204 and 232 tips, you've chosen to do between 71 and 80 percent of the suggestions in this book.

- If you checked off between 233 and 261 tips, you've chosen to do between 81 and 90 percent of the suggestions in this book.

- If you checked off between 262 and 288 tips, you've chosen to do between 91 and 100 percent of the suggestions in this book.

YOUR FINAL RESULTS

Drum roll please—ladies and gentlemen, the moment you've all been waiting for has arrived. It's time to analyze your point score and see how you measure up. Then we'll utilize your tip percentage to help guide you to improving your results—if that's necessary. It very well may not be.

WHAT YOUR POINT TOTAL SAYS

1 TO 199 POINTS

Hmmm—this is a low score. I'm not going to kid you, I'm not thrilled. If you fall into this point range, it tells me something critical—that you're inconsistent with your level of commitment to yourself and to your health and well-being. Even if you marked off every tip in Chapters 1 and 2, which are the essential ingredients for weight loss, you have neglected incorporating the tips in the other chapters. This gives a huge disconnect, as the lower-ranked tips exist to help you implement the tips in the first two chapters. Or maybe it's the opposite; maybe you've marked off many of the lower-ranked tips in Chapters 3 to 7 but have not committed enough to the overall weight-loss concepts supplied in Chapters 1 and 2. Even worse, possibly you haven't devoted yourself enough across the board, failing to select enough tips overall and too few quality suggestions to get this score. Regardless, the implication is the same: inconsistency and a failure to truly commit and/or truly implement.

Believe it or not, there's good news: something is better than nothing. If you're in this point range, you won't continue gaining weight. That's a good thing—a really good thing. The actions you have decided to take will kill any chance that you'll take in more calories than you're burning. However, whether you lose weight and get the slim, sexy body you bought this book for is questionable. If you do lose weight, the rate will be slow. If you're lucky, you'll shed a pound every 1 or 2 weeks. With this level of commitment, I also question whether you'll keep it off.

I don't want to discourage you. You still deserve that pat on the back for attempting to change how you take care of you. But let this serve as a wake-up call. Why did you buy this book? Are you willing and ready to take responsibility and do more? Because you *can* do more.

To move the needle forward—or rather backward, where the scale is concerned—we need to evaluate your tip percentage, then make some adjustments according to where you fall.

- If you've committed to over 50 percent of the tips in the book, then you need to go back and choose more of the power tips, aka the 3-pointers in Chapters 1, 2, and 3.
- Conversely, if you're under 50 percent but are on the high end of this score range, it tells me you've selected many of the power tips. Now you need to give some serious thought to how you're going to implement them to solidify your slim lifestyle. You specifically need to revisit Chapters 4 and 6 and get real about where your slim might be sabotaged. You need to arm yourself and plan ahead if you expect to stick with the tips in the earlier chapters.
- If you're under 50 percent and on the lower end of this score range, you need a do-over! Go back to Chapters 1, 2, 3, 4, 5, and 6 and add at least four tips from each of these chapters that you feel you can truly commit to in your daily life.

200 TO 350 POINTS

Okay, while I'm hoping you're on the higher end of this point spread, overall this isn't a bad category to fall into score-wise. It shows me that you get the idea and that you see how to connect the dots that lead to slim. The general principles that lead to a slim lifestyle are amenable to you, and you're willing to do enough to implement them successfully. This range is not going to get you the quickest results, but you'll get results, and that's what matters most. My one concern if you fall in this range is that if you don't see a fast enough body transformation, you may get discouraged.

If you want to move at a quicker pace, here's what I recommend:

- If your tip percentage is between 30 to 50 percent, it shows me you've selected more 2- and 3-pointers overall, which is a good thing, but I highly suggest you add *more tips in general*. Revisit Chapter 5 and give some consideration to what will get you psyched and incentivized to dig a little deeper. Aim to add at least 20 points here. Also, take another glance at Chapters 3 and 4 to see where you might shore up your slim approach with some simple but effective 1-pointers in Slim Cheffing, Slim Dining, and Eats at the Office.
- If your tip percentage is between 50 and 70 percent, it would seem, based on your total point score and your tip percentage, that you have chosen a nice cross-section of tips from all chapters in all point ranges. To up the ante here, I want you to try to add 10 points from each of Chapters 1,2, 3, 4, and 7. This will add a little more action overall to your plan and really accelerate your results.
- Now, if you're at 70 percent tip utilization, you're definitely on the higher end of this spectrum. If you fall into this category, it tells me you've chosen many of the tips with a lower point allotment. You need to add some fitness power tips—some 3-pointers—stat. Head straight over to Chapter 2, and add as many of the "Maximize Your Muscle" and "Amp Up Your Cardio" tips as you can.
- Again, you aren't in bad shape if you've ended up in this category, but to enhance and accelerate your results, follow my outlined recommendations above.

351 TO 450 POINTS

Now this score makes me happy. Truly. This is the ideal spot. While you may have thought that getting the highest point score was ideal, the truth is that living this way may not be sustainable or realistic to your everyday life. Landing within this point range tells me that you have a solid understanding of what slim requires and you're willing to put in the work, but you're sensible and grounded with what you can fit in and maintain permanently. Getting this score means you have selected not only enough tips but many of the power tips, so that you get escalated, transformational, and lasting results.

If you fall on the higher end of this point score (401 to 450), don't change a thing! You're in a great spot poised for success! For those of you who fall on the lower end of this range (351 to 400), and are looking to up the ante a tad and add some finishing touches, here's what you should do:

- If your tip percentage is 40 percent or less, you could go back to Chapters 3 and 4 and add 5 to 10 more tips per chapter. This is to make sure you've retained enough strategies to apply the general slim principles outlined in Chapters 1 and 2.
- In addition, take a quick swing past Chapter 5 to make sure your motivation is firmly established. I would aim to check at least one-third of the tips in this chapter to make your continued plan of attack ironclad.
- If your tip percentage is 40 to 80 percent, you've chosen a decent number of ideas that run the gamut in point allowance. I propose you review Chapter 6 to make sure you've truly conquered this material. Remember, you can work out and eat right, but if you constantly cave to hunger and cravings, your results will slow. If something unforeseen comes along and knocks you for a loop, it's imperative that you be prepared to jump right back on the horse. Also, be sure to

swing by Chapter 7 once more and play with some of these supercharged tips. They'll help you maximize your results and the time in which you attain them.

450 TO 613 POINTS

Liar. No, seriously, are you this hard-core? I don't even fall into this bracket. This is some serious commitment, and it can only mean that you have an insanely high tip percentage *and* you chose nearly all the power tips. I'm stoked for you, superimpressed, and have no advice for you to better your results. But I do have a brief word of caution. While I love your gusto, if you land in the higher range of this range, above 500, be wary not to fall into an all-or-nothing mentality. This extreme resolve is very hard to maintain.

I'm worried you might be obsessing too much about your slim lifestyle. When you slip a bit (and you will, we all do, no one's perfect all the time), I'm concerned that you may freak out, get discouraged, and give up. I've known many a dieter who started out 100 percent in and then got exhausted and overwhelmed and consequently gave up entirely. They just couldn't keep up such an oppressive level of commitment. Plus, if you're too regimented, life is just no damn fun.

Remember my promise back on page 1? I swore I'd get you amazing results without making you miserable. Here's my advice: I love that most of the tips seem doable to you, but consider allowing yourself some leniency. Remember to live by the 80/20 rule. You're going to really need that 20 percent of reprieve to sustain this agenda and maintain your sanity.

For example, I hardly ever drink, but once in a while I do have a margarita with my pals. Another example: I follow all the tips on how to maximize my muscles, but there are weeks I'm so crazed, I get to the gym only once. It happens. Take a breath and just know that it's okay to cut yourself a little slack. It's also okay to fall outside the lines from to time to time. If you can work all these tips in 80 percent of the time, you'll still get amazing results without getting burned out.

NO TIP LEFT BEHIND

At the beginning of the book, I suggested that you pick and choose tips that both resonate with you and are manageable with your lifestyle. What do you do about the tips you didn't choose? Keep 'em in the idea bank and withdraw them later. Over the next few months, stick with what you've chosen, live with them, experience them, and see the results these ideas bring you. Then after a bit, you can go back through the chapters and tweak accordingly: exchange tips out if need be, or add a few more to your arsenal to maintain a decent point score.

I don't want this book to be a once-read, I want you to reread it and use it over and over as often as you need to for its information and for reassurance. With it, you can keep the special combination that belongs only to you, one that cracks the code of how to get and stay slim for life.

SEE YA, SLIM

Well, here we are, at the end of the book, but it's the beginning of your slim life. By living, truly living, this information, you've essentially bulletproofed your path to slim. I promise, you now know everything you need to get the results you want, and in a timeframe that will keep you encouraged. Knowledge is power. Now you have it. Empowered, you're capable of taking the effective actions that will yield the change you want and deserve.

As you've probably noticed by now, *Slim for Life* isn't really a diet book. Diet books are often about spending a few weeks or months doing something you won't want to keep doing later or over the long term. Instead, it's a book that teaches you a new way of life, a far happier and much *slimmer* way. One where you're never again confused or lost about what to do to get a slim, sexy physique and stay on top of your health. The days of being duped by fad diets, ripped off by worthless fitness gadgets (hello Shake Weight), scammed by pharmaceutical companies pushing dangerous drugs, or harmed by life-threatening surgeries are over. You know better now, and because of this, *no one* can f* with you ever again. (I went the whole book without dropping the f-bomb, but I couldn't help myself here. Damn editor cleaned it up.)

I mean it. No one can mess with you, Slim.

If you ever doubt it, don't forget that I've *never* met a person I couldn't get weight off of. Everything I do with my own body and health is in this book, as well as everything I've ever done and implemented to get radical results in the thousands of others I've helped to find their slim.

Now go kick some ass (your own preferably) and wow yourself. You got this!

SELECTED REFERENCES

JOURNAL ARTICLES

Behm, D. G., and A. Chaouachi. "A Review of the Acute Effects of Static and Dynamic Stretching on Performance." *European Journal of Applied Physiology* 111, no. 11 (2011): 2633–51. Epub 2011 Mar 4.

Børsheim, E., and R. Bahr. "Effect of Exercise Intensity, Duration and Mode on Post-Exercise Oxygen Consumption." *Sports Medicine* 33, no. 14 (2003): 1037–60.

Broom, D. R., et al. "Influence of Resistance and Aerobic Exercise on Hunger, Circulating Levels of Acylated Ghrelin, and Peptide YY in Healthy Males." *American Journal of Physiology* 296, no. 1 (2009): R29-R35.

Burgomaster, K. A., et al. "Similar Metabolic Adaptations During Exercise After Low Volume Sprint Interval and Traditional Endurance Training in Humans." *Journal of Physiology* 586, no. 1 (2008): 151–60. Epub 2007 Nov 8.

Burleson, M. A., et al. "Effect of Weight Training Exercise and Treadmill Exercise on Elevated Post-Exercise Oxygen Consumption." *Medicine and Science in Sports and Exercise* 30 (1998): 518–22.

Carlson, O., et al. "Impact of Reduced Meal Frequency Without Caloric Restriction on Glucose Regulation in Healthy, Normal-Weight Middle-Aged Men and Women." *Metabolism* 56, no. 12 (2007): 1729–34.

Daussin, F. N., et al. "Effect of Interval Versus Continuous Training on Cardiorespiratory and Mitochondrial Functions: Relationship to Aerobic Performance Improvements in Sedentary Subjects." *American Journal of Physiology: Regulatory, Integrative and Comparative Physiology* 295 (2008): R264–72.

Dyck, D. J. "Leptin Sensitivity in Skeletal Muscle Is Modulated by Diet and Exercise." *Exercise Sport Science Reviews* 33, no. 4 (2005): 189–94.

Elliot, D. L., et al. "Effect of Resistance Training on Excess Post-Exercise Oxygen Consumption." *Journal of Applied Sport Science Research* 6, no. 2 (1992): 77–81.

Evero, N., et al. "Aerobic Exercise Reduces Neuronal Responses in Food Reward Brain Regions." *Journal of Applied Physiology* 112, no. 9 (2012): 1612–19. Epub 2012 Mar 1.

Finlayson, G. "Low Fat Loss Response After Medium-Term Supervised Exercise in Obese Is Associated with Exercise-Induced Increase in Food Reward." *Journal of Obesity* 2011 (2011). doi:10.1155/2011/615624. Epub 2010 Sep 20.

Hall, C., et al. "Energy Expenditure of Walking and Running: Comparison with Prediction Equations." *Medicine and Science in Sports and Exercise* 36, no. 12 (2004): 2128–34.

Hall, Kevin D., et al. "Quantification of the Effect of Energy Imbalance on Bodyweight." *Lancet* 378, no. 9793 (2011): 826–37. http://www.thelancet.com/journals/lancet/article/PIIS0140-6736%2811%2960812-X/abstract.

Haltom, R. W., et al. "Circuit Weight Training and Its Effects on Excess Post Exercise Oxygen Consumption." *Medicine and Science in Sports and Exercise* 31 (1999): 1613–18.

Heden, T., et al. "One-Set Resistance Training Elevates Energy Expenditure for 72 H Similar to Three Sets." *European Journal of Applied Physiology* 111, no. 3 (2011): 477–84.

Helgerud, J., et al. "Aerobic High-Intensity Intervals Improve VO2max More Than Moderate Training." *Medicine and Science in Sports and Exercise* 39, no. 4 (2007): 665–71.

Knab, A. M., et al. "A 45-Minute Vigorous Exercise Bout Increases Metabolic Rate for 14 Hours." *Medicine and Science in Sports and Exercise* 43, no. 9 (2011): 1643–48.

Kohler, J. J., et al. "Muscle Activation Patterns While Lifting Stable and Unstable Loads on Stable and Unstable Surfaces." *Journal of Strength and Conditioning Research* 24, no. 2 (2010): 313–21.

Kravitz, L. "Resistance Training: Adaptations and Health Implications." *IDEA Today* 14, no. 9 (1996): 38–46.

———. "New Insights Into Circuit Training." *IDEA Fitness Journal* 2, no. 4 (2005): 24–26.

———. "Aerobic and Resistance Training Sequence." *IDEA Fitness Journal* 4, no. 4 (2007): 20–21.

Melby, C., et al. "Effect of Acute Resistance Exercise on Post-Exercise Energy Expenditure and Resting Metabolic Rate." *Journal of Applied Physiology* 75 (1993): 1847–53.

Peterson, J. M., et al. "Ibuprofen and Acetaminophen: Effect on Muscle Inflammation After Eccentric Exercise." *Medicine and Science in Sports and Exercise* 35, no. 6 (2003): 892–96.

Samson, M., et al. "Effects of Dynamic and Static Stretching Within General and Activity Specific Warm-Up Protocols." *Journal of Sports Science and Medicine* 11 (2012): 279-85, http://www.jssm.org/vol11/n2/11/v11n2-11pdf.pdf.

Spennewyn, K. C. "Strength Outcomes in Fixed Versus Free-Form Resistance Equipment." *Journal of Strength and Conditioning Research* 22, no. 1 (2008): 75–81.

Tabata, I., et al. "Effects of Moderate-Intensity Endurance and High-Intensity Intermittent Training on Anaerobic Capacity and VO2max." *Medicine and Science in Sports and Exercise* 28, no. 10 (1996): 1327–30.

Talanian, J., et al. "Two Weeks of High-Intensity Aerobic Interval Training Increases the Capacity for Fat Oxidation During Exercise in Women." *Journal of Applied Physiology* 102, no. 4 (2007): 1439-47.

Trapp, E. G., et al. "The Effects of High-Intensity Intermittent Exercise Training on Fat Loss and Fasting Insulin Levels of Young Women." *International Journal of Obesity* 32, no. 4 (2008): 684–91.

Wilkin, L. D. "Energy Expenditure Comparison Between Walking and Running in Average Fitness Individuals." *Journal of Strength and Conditioning Research* 26, no. 4 (2012): 1039–44.

OTHER REFERENCES

"The Best Diet Is the One You'll Follow." Harvard School of Public Health, November 11, 2012, http://www.hsph.harvard.edu/nutritionsource/healthy-weight/best-weight-loss-diet/.

Brody, Jane E. "An Oldie Vies for Nutrient of the Decade," February 19, 2008, http://www.nytimes.com/2008/02/19/health/19brod.html?_r=0.

Carolyn_r. "Does Exercise Make You Eat Less or More?" Healthy Eating Blog on Calorie Count, May 2, 2012, http://caloriecount.about.com/does-exercise-make-you-eat-less-b568816.

"Confirmed Again: Statin Drugs Accelerate Cardiovascular Disease." *Food Consumer,* October 15, 2012, http://www.foodconsumer.org/newsite/Non-food/Drug/statin_drugs_accelerate_cardiovascular_disease_1015120825.html.

Connealy, Leigh Erin, M.D. "Aspartame: Is the Sweet Taste Worth the Harm?" *Food Matters,* April 28, 2010, http://www.foodmatters.tv/articles-1/aspartame-is-the-sweet-taste-worth-the-harm.

"Exercise Reduces Hunger in Lean Women but Not Obese Women." Endocrine Society, November 6, 2012, http://www.endo-society.org/media/ENDO-08/research/Exercise-reduces-hunger-in-lean-women.cfm.

"Fat Epidemic Linked to Chemicals Run Amok." MSNBC, March 8, 2010, http://www.msnbc.msn.com/id/35315651/ns/health-diet_and_nutrition/t/fat-epidemic-linked-chemicals-run-amok/#.UKAJy9UU-So.

Gorman, Megan Othersen. "A New Study Found That Just as Food Odors Can Trigger Hunger, Food Odors Can Also Activate Areas of the Brain That Trigger the Feeling of Fullness." *Rodale,* November 2011, http://www.rodale.com/appetite-control.

Haupt, Angela. "Food and Mood: 6 Ways Your Diet Affects How You Feel." *U.S. News & World Report*, August 31, 2011, http://health.usnews.com/health-news/diet-fitness/diet/articles/2011/08/31/food-and-mood-6-ways-your-diet-affects-how-you-feel.

Hopf, Sarah-Marie."You Are What You Eat: How Food Affects Your Mood." *Dartmouth Undergraduate Journal of Science*, 2010, http://dujs.dartmouth.edu/fall-2010/you-are-what-you-eat-how-food-affects-your-mood.

"How the Smell of Food Affects How Much You Eat." *Science Daily*, March 19, 2012, http://www.sciencedaily.com/releases/2012/03/120321094137.htm.

"Inflammatory Pathway Genes Belong to Major Targets of Persistent Organic Pollutants in Adipose Cells." *Environmental Health Perspectives* 120, no. 4 (2012): 508–14. doi: 10.1289/ehp.1104282, PMCID: PMC3339464. Epub January 19, 2012.

"Is There Any Nutritional Difference Between Wild-Caught and Farm-Raised Fish? Is One Type Better for Me than the Other?" George Mateljan Foundation, 2010, http://www.whfoods.com/genpage.php?tname=george&dbid=96.

Jennings, Trent. "Does Your Body Burn More Calories if You Are Hot or if You Are Cold?" *Livestrong*, August 24, 2011, http://www.livestrong.com/article/526014-does-your-body-burn-more-calories-if-you-are-hot-or-if-you-are-cold/#ixzz2BxxBz5Y9.

Krieger, Ellie. "Bigger Portions of the Right Foods Can Help Dieters." *USA Today*, September 18, 2012, http://usatoday30.usatoday.com/news/nation/story/2012/09/18/bigger-portions-of-the-right-foods-can-help-dieters/57802742/1.

Larson, Nicole I., et al. "Making Time for Meals: Meal Structure and Associations with Dietary Intake in Young Adults." *Journal of the American Dietetic Association* 109, no. 1 (2009).

Leong, Kristie, M.D. "Does Drinking Cold Water Burn Calories,?" *Yahoo Voices*, May 10, 2010, http://voices.yahoo.com/does-drinking-cold-water-burn-calories-5994106.html?cat=51.

Main, Emily. "Your Allergy Meds Could Be Making You Fat." *Women's Health Magazine*, May 15, 2012, http://www.womenshealthmag.com/health/allergy-side-effects.

"Mood-food Connection: We Eat More and Less-Healthy Comfort Foods When We Feel Down, Study Finds," *Cornell University Chronicle*, January 23, 2007, http://www.news.cornell.edu/stories/Jan07/food.mood.sl.html.

"Morning Workout Benefits Include Curbing Appetite and More," *Huffington Post*, September 12, 2012, http://www.huffingtonpost.com/2012/09/20/morning-workouts-curb-appetite_n_1900889.html.

"New Almond Study Finds Chewing Is More than Meets the Mouth: Thorough Chewing," Reuters, May 7, 2009, http://www.reuters.com/article/2009/05/07/idUS212878+07-May-2009+PRN20090507.

"NSAIDs (Ibuprofen, Acetaminophen/Paracetamol) for Runners, Impairs Healing and Interferes with Hydration," August 19, 2011, http://fellrnr.com/wiki/NSAIDs_and_Running.

"Obesogens: An Environmental Link to Obesity." *Environmental Health Perspectives*, U.S. National Library of Health, National Institutes of Health, February 2012, http://www.ncbi.nlm.nih.gov/pmc/articles/PMC3279464/.

O'Calaghan, Tiffany. "Study: Quick Weight Loss May Yield Lasting Results." *Time*, May 6, 2010, http://healthland.time.com/2010/05/06/study-quick-weight-loss-may-yield-lasting-results/#ixzz2ByKKZvDG.

Parker-Pope, Tara. "The Risks and Rewards of Skipping Meals." *New York Times*, December 26, 2007, http://well.blogs.nytimes.com/2007/12/26/the-risks-and-rewards-of-skipping-meals/.

"Research Summary: Dairy and Healthy Weight," National Dairy Council, 2012, http://www.nationaldairycouncil.org/Research/ResearchSummaries/Pages/DairyandHealthyWeightResearchSummary.aspx.

Sawyers, Mary. "CHR Study Finds Keeping Food Diaries Doubles Weight Loss." Center for Health Research, July 8, 2008, http://www.kpchr.org/research/public/News.aspx?NewsID=3.

"The Secrets to Weight Loss: Keep a Food Journal, Don't Skip Meals, Eat In." *Time*, July 13, 2012, http://healthland.time.com/2012/07/13/the-secrets-to-weight-loss-keep-a-food-journal-dont-skip-meals-eat-in/#ixzz2BwmXeV7k.

Shy, Leta. "Comment on 'Why Exercise Makes You Eat More,'" *Fitsugar Blog*, April 18, 2012, http://www.fitsugar.com/Why-Exercise-Makes-You-Eat-More-22721812#comments.

Song, Sora. "What Does a Clean House Have to Do with Health?" *Time*, June 2, 2010.

Springen, Karen. "Pets: Good for Your Health?" *Daily Beast*, January 10, 2008, http://www.thedailybeast.com/newsweek/2008/01/10/pets-good-for-your-health.html.

"Vacations Provide Mental Health Benefits for Women," *Marshfield Clinic*, November 28, 2005, http://www.marshfieldclinic.org/patients/?page=newsreleases&id=2831.

Warren, Ellen. "You'll Buy Less Junk Food If You Pay in Cash." *Chicago Tribune*, January 25, 2012, http://articles.chicagotribune.com/2012-01-25/health/sc-health-0125-bit-of-fit-20120125_1_junk-food-credit-card-cash.

"When 3,500 Calories Do Not Equal a Pound: New Study," *Stone Hearth News*, August 26, 2011, http://www.stonehearthnewsletters.com/when-3500-calories-do-not-equal-a-pound-new-study/exercise/.

"A Widely Used, Understudied Chemical Alters Inflammation." *Environmental Health News*, December 12, 2008, http://www.environmentalhealthnews.org/ehs/newscience/a-widely-used-understudied-chemical-alters-inflammation.

Wilcox, Christie. "Understanding Our Bodies: Serotonin, the Connection Between Food and Mood." *Nutrition Wonderland*, June 24, 2009, http://nutritionwonderland.com/2009/06/understanding-bodies-serotonin-connection-between-food-and-mood/.

Woodward, M., and H. Tunstall-Pedoe. "Coffee and Tea Consumption in the Scottish Heart Health Study Follow Up: Conflicting Relations with Coronary Risk Factors, Coronary Disease, and All Cause Mortality." *Journal of Epidemiological and Community Health* 53 (1999): 481–87, doi:10.1136/jech.53.8.481.

"Yogurt Increases Fat Loss, UT Study Shows," *Tennessee Today*, University of Tennessee, April 14, 2003, http://www.utk.edu/tntoday/2003/04/14/yogurt-increases-fat-loss-ut-study-shows/.

Zerbe, Leah. "Does This Chemical Make Me Look Fat? 'Obesogens' Lurk All Around Us," *Rodale*, February 24, 2012, http://www.rodale.com/obesogens.

ACKNOWLEDGMENTS

Special thanks to my incredible team of badasses at Empowered Media: Ray, Julie, Danny, Autumn, Brittany, and Erica. They work tirelessly to make the world a better place—especially my business partner Giancarlo Chersich. You are a dear friend and my most trusted comrade in arms.

To my tireless and extremely patient editor, Heather Jackson, who has guided me swiftly and successfully time and time again with truth and excellence.

To Crown Publishing and the Archetype and Harmony Books team for always having my back.

To my talented and wise consigliere and writing partner, Linda Shelton.

To my fearless lawyer, David Markman.

To my partners at Everyday Health who power jillianmichaels.com.

And of course to my beautiful family: Heidi, Lu, and Phoenix. Thank you for your love and support. You are my heart always.

INDEX

Note: Page numbers in *italics* refer to recipes.

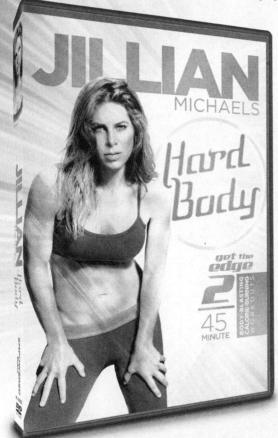
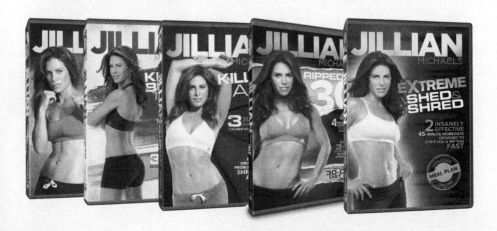